CHAKRAS –
RAYS AND RADIONICS

by

DAVID V. TANSLEY D.C.

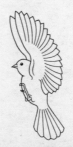

SAFFRON WALDEN
THE C.W. DANIEL COMPANY LIMITED

First published in Great Britain
by the C. W. Daniel Company Limited,
1 Church Path, Saffron Walden, Essex, England

4th Impression 1988

ISBN 0 85207 161 2

Set in 10/11 point Bembo by Simpson Typesetting,
Bishop's Stortford, Herts, England.
and printed by Hillman Printers (Frome) Ltd., Somerset, England

This book is dedicated to
The Radionic Practitioners of the Future

ACKNOWLEDGEMENTS

I wish to acknowledge my debt to The Lucis Press: London, for use of material from the writings of Alice A. Bailey, in particular *Esoteric Healing, Esoteric Psychology, Vols. I and II., Discipleship in the New Age, A Treatise on Cosmic Fire* and *A Treatise on White Magic*. For without the principles laid down in her books, none of my own writings would have been possible. I also wish to acknowledge the use of material drawn from *Esoteric Healing – Flower Remedies and Esoteric Astrology* by Dr Douglas Baker, B.A., M.R.C.S., L.R.C.P., F.Z.S. *The 7 Temperaments of Man* by Geoffrey Hodson, Theosophical Publishing House, Madras. *The Seven Rays of Energy* by Michal Eastcott, Sundial House. *The Flower Essence Quarterly,* Richard Katz, Editor. Nevada City, California. *Flower Essences* by Gurudas, published by Brotherhood of Life, Albuquerque, New Mexico. I would like to put on record too, my appreciation for the posthumous contribution on the miasms by the late John Damonte. And my thanks to Tad Mann who is responsible for the design of the cover on this book, my radionic analysis charts, and much more. I would like to record here my gratitude to Rosemary Russell who has been a constant source of encouragement, particularly over the past twelve months. I would also like to take this opportunity to thank Phyllis and Leslie Speight, who in 1972, against all advice published *Radionics and the Subtle Anatomy of Man*. It has now gone into five editions and given rise to the rest of my books in this field. My thanks to Ian Miller who continues to publish my radionic books, ship them, and even fly half way round the world to unpack them and place them on the shelves. Seldom has an author had such service, given so freely and with such humour.

PREFACE

On the morning of Wednesday, March 7th 1984 I sat down at the typewriter and drafted a seven page synopsis of a book on healing, which I duly submitted to a publisher. By the afternoon I knew that another book was 'imminent' sitting complete in Dimension II. I knew that it was to be a book dealing with the ray energies in radionics, and I knew that it would be my last book on the subject of radionics, completing my contribution to this field. I returned to my typewriter and finished the manuscript for this book within the space of fifty-five hours of typing time – first draft being the final draft. The book had not been planned; like *Radionics: Science or Magic?* it knocked on the door of my consciousness and demanded expression at a time when I was not only overloaded with work, but beginning the process of moving house. It had also been preceded by the writing of two other books *The Raiment of Light* and *Radionics: A Patients Guide*.

I am relating these facts here because this phenomena fascinates me. It happened with three previous books, *Omens of Awareness, Dimensions of Radionics* and *Radionics: Science or Magic?* The three books I wrote prior to *Omens of Awareness* were sheer drudgery and required much correction and rewriting. Why this has changed I do not know, but an explanation would seem to lie in the theories outlined in *Radionics: Science or Magic?* and the excellent books by Jane Roberts, in respect to Dimensions I and II. I can only theorise that an alignment takes place between my right and left mind-brain hemispheres, and perhaps between the higher aspects of my mental body and the buddhic plane – I don't know what the mechanics of the phenomena are, but I do know that these books make their appearance as a constant stream of words and ideas, some of which I have never considered before. My energy levels are very high and I inevitably wake at 3 a.m. or earlier, get up and begin work. I seldom feel tired from this work but my physical body drops weight which I can ill afford to lose.

No doubt my writing style and use of the English language leaves a lot to be desired, but this does not concern me too much as the purpose of these books is to present ideas for other people to use, and primarily it seems, to give radionics a new direction; which it has taken since *Radionics and the Subtle Anatomy of Man* was first published in 1972.

In *Chakras — Rays and Radionics* lies the key to a whole new approach to this field of healing and distant treatment. These principles demand that practitioners acquire a deeper understanding of the chakras, subtle bodies, and especially of the rays in order to render themselves effective in their chosen field of service.

I hope that this book and my previous volumes on radionics will provide a stepping off point and a platform for those presently practicing radionics, and a guide to those in the future who enter this work better equipped to carry it forward into the 21st century, than we are.

Uppark Estate, Sussex. March 1984

CONTENTS

ILLUSTRATIONS

INTRODUCTION

Ten years ago, in 1974 I became acquainted for the first time with *Radionics and the Subtle Anatomy of Man,* by David Tansley. Since then I have read all of his books eagerly, including *Omens of Awareness.* My fascination for his writings lay as much with the content as with the style and expressiveness of the man behind the words. I enjoyed his sense of humour which I think is always a characteristic of anything true, combined with a refreshing mixture of spirituality and down-to-earthness. Here was somebody who knew what he was talking about, and who was at home with a whole range of different 'languages' – the medical language, the radionic language and the language of the esoteric teachings – and who realised at the same time that all of this knowledge only reflects a small aspect of the unnameable Unity. Here to my mind was someone who worked in a magical as well as mystical way, an important ability in the healing arts.

This gave me a strong feeling of affinity with Tansley. I was working in a similar manner but in a different area. As a Psycho-therapist (one language) I was helping people to get back to their Source (another language), and because of this I began to use a variety of energy based techniques (again another language). I was seeking in this way to integrate within myself and within my work, the psychological language of Freud, Jung and Fritz Perls with the esoteric language of the gnostics, alchemists and the mystics and the 'energy language' of Wilhelm Reich and Alexander Lowen. This fusion meant an enormous increase in the breadth and depth of each one of the separate 'languages', but I too experienced the tremendous difficulties of creating a synthesis, and the inner stresses that accompany such a task often left me wondering where I belonged, and if the task was one that could be accomplished in practical terms.

It became clear over the years as I read Tansley's books that they formed a sequential picture of his own growth and understanding of the healing process. What intrigued me was – would he finally succeed in explaining the phenomenon of radionics and the role that the apparatus played in distant diagnosis and treatment. These questions connect very directly with my own professional territory where I ask them in a wider sense. What is healing really about, how is it caused – if indeed it is possible to use the word caused in respect to healing – and by what means is it served?

Whilst on holiday in 1983 at a Mediterranean resort I read *Radionics: Science or Magic?* This book clarified the above questions for me, and I understood at that point, Tansley's answer. Properly speaking we are a Unity. This is the basis of our wholeness and the point from which we heal. The problem is that we do not realise our wholeness and function in a cloud of unknowing. For this reason we create forms and apparatus such as radionic instruments to help us deal with our lack of knowledge and understanding of the energies and inner processes that are involved. Healing, Tansley appeared to be saying, was not something that happened in our space/time reality but is related to the Wholeness which is outside of space/time. Contact with the Wholeness brings healing, instantly. Faith is the channel which introduces it into the space/time reality. In other words it is not so much a matter of 'vibrations' as a subtler spiritual process.

I heaved a sigh of relief when I read this because over the years I had come to the same conclusion in my own work. In reality little or nothing is accomplished by the rituals, the sessions, the working on complex mother and father images or dreams. These are the forms we need to believe we can change, that by manipulating them we can let the Light into our existence. In reality the Light is there, it simply requires recognition. As we realise this we begin to abandon the 'importance' of the technique, we let go of the apparatus to participate in the Unity. As a personality I heal nobody, healing does not take place from me to the client in my consulting room. It happens when I let the Spirit move me, in this manner I need less and less external apparatus and ritual because I become more and more of an instrument through my service to others.

I resolved after reading *Radionics: Science or Magic?* to get in touch with the author upon my return to Holland. This happened in a way I had not envisaged – I fell ill with a serious throat inflammation and completely lost my voice. At the same time a whole series of adverse events entered my life, and I experienced a heavy sense of physical and mental oppression. It was one of the darkest valleys I have been through in my life. I knew that I had to meditate and reflect instead of letting my reactive feelings get the best of me, I knew that I had to stay connected at all costs with my deepest knowledge, with my Inner Guide. This was the real struggle and I knew then that I had to ask for help, a help different from that given by my doctor, wife or friends. For this reason I wrote to David Tansley asking him to help me with my physical condition and to aid me in remaining connected to my Self.

His answer came rapidly and it came as a shock. The content of my radionic analysis threw me into a deep turmoil. I was no longer the only one who saw how serious the situation was. Paradoxically the analysis gave me a sense of rest and something to hold onto. This particularly applied to the description of my ray makeup which clearly defined my life-task and potentials as well as the problems that accompany them. At my request Tansley advised me as to which homoeopathic remedies I should take, and proceeded to treat me radionically. While these of course proved very helpful, by far the greatest help was derived from his description of my rays. My ray profile provided me with a specific framework with which to align my questions and problems, also my feelings and thoughts in respect to my central life-task.

I was not altogether unfamiliar with the Language of the rays. Thiry years previous, as a young boy, I had read many of the books written by Alice Bailey. Like many people I found them difficult to come to grips with, nevertheless they fascinated me and over the years I read and studied them from time to time. Gradually I became more familiar with this fundamental way of looking at things, but it was not yet possible for these thoughts to take root in my life. While the rays interested me, their qualites were so archetypal that I could see all of their many qualities in myself. This made it difficult if not virtually impossible for me to deliniate my own rays. The fact that Tansley named and described my ray-constellation for me made it possible to meditate in accordance with myself during this crisis period in my life, fostering fresh nourishment and giving new impetus to the study of this material which will involve me for a long time to come, just as it has engrossed me in the past. In this manner the old didactic law that the best way for the pupil to absorb knowledge is to apply it directly to his own life-situation, became true for me.

Over quite a number of years now I have trained and educated people in the spiritual and psychological sciences. Working with groups in Holland and Germany, bringing them to an awareness of their own Source and how best to employ themselves in service. The people that form these groups come from all areas of commerce and industry and they include physicians, judges, psychotherapists, economists and healers. They are all characterized by their skill in at least one profession (one language) and by the fact that they want to put this skill to use in service to the Greater Whole. Each of them wants to do more than the contractual demands placed upon them by their profession. I help them to realise this ability, and that is why I call this group work, 'Training in Helpership'. We accept in the group that each of us has his or her own qualities, and that these can become distorted when employed to serve the ends of the little ego. This distortion leads eventually to crisis points, so I consider it essential that participants become familiar with their core-qualities and the distortions that are manifesting in them.

The moment I received Tansley's radionic analysis with the description of my ray qualities, and experienced the benefits of the insight it provided I realized that the teaching of the rays was of the greatest importance to my training groups. Here was the ultimate framework in which all of the other systems could find their place – the connective tissue that would bring them all together.

Tansley then made a full radionic analysis for each member of one of my training groups, and we worked with this material during a three day seminar. I filled in the background for them by teaching the theory of the rays, and we then began to engage ourselves specifically with the ray-configurations of individual members and exploring the effects of these rays in the relationships that existed between various members of the group. It was quite remarkable how relationships could be clarified in this manner, basing our observations and insights on the ray energies.

In this particular group it transpired that half of the members had a transpersonal self on the second ray, which perhaps is not surprising when you consider that they were seeking to serve in the deepest sense of the word, through their chosen profession. A similar number were found to have their mental body upon the fifth ray which was in keeping with their interest in the study of esoteric psychology. It was no coincidence, that I as leader of the group also had a second ray transpersonal self and a fifth ray mental body, which both served as focal point of specific energies to which the group was drawn. Our work with the rays enabled us to throw much light on the struggles and disagreements of various group members, as well as to explore and experience the harmonies and sympathies from the point of view of the different rays involved. It was obvious that here was a whole area of exploration of self that had lain fallow, and one I intend to investigate in the coming years. One such area is marriage counselling – the use of ray configurations would provide a most useful insight into the way partners interact and conduct their relationship. From my own personal experience of using the ray energy qualities it is evident that they are a key to far deeper insights than had heretofore been available in respect to the nature of man and his response to life.

Chakras – Rays and Radionics provides the basic information upon which therapists can build – the book is a key-stone for use by practitioners, not only of radionics but in the fields of social work, psychotherapy, medicine and healing. As such I strongly recommend it to those who have the courage to extend their vision and offer their uniqueness in service to the One who is guiding us.

Hans Korteweg.

CHAPTER ONE

BOUNDARIES AND BARRIERS

Growth fundamentally means an enlarging and expanding of one's horizons, a growth of one's boundaries, outwardly in perspective and inwardly in depth.

No Boundary – Ken Wilbur

In the proceedings of the Scientific and Technical Congress of Radionics and Radiesthesia held in London on May 16th-18th 1950, the Reverend Paul W. Eardley in his introduction to the lecturer Ronald Thornton, D.Sc., Ph.D., said,

Firstly, although this is, rightly, a scientific gathering, the philosophical, metaphysical and – dare I say it? – theological implications of our deliberations are quite tremendous.

Since the 1950's radionics has expanded its horizons and deepened its perspectives, pushing back the limiting boundaries and barriers that were implicit in its rather physical approach. Today the language and terminology of physical medicine, anatomy and physiology is complemented by a more metaphysical parlance – we now speak of the subtle anatomy, the chakras and the ray energies which form and qualify the outer man. Disease, while recognised in orthodox terms, is seen to arise from particular energy imbalances in the chakras or subtle bodies themselves. In 1950 radionic practitioners did not determine the states of the chakras, today it is common practice. Nor did they ascertain the conditions present in the subtle bodies as such, but now they do – these aspects of diagnosis which have radically altered the face of radionics over the past decade simply were not used in the earlier years, and yet if the Reverend Eardley's statement is anything to go by, the potential was there, just waiting to be expressed.

The fact is, radionics is a healing art without limit, its potential is the potential of the human mind and the human power to heal. The only limitation that can be placed on it, is that of the individual practitioner's knowledge and quality of awareness. It might help to examine this idea a little more closely because it is vitally important to fully understand what is involved.

Curiously enough we need boundaries and barriers, we need the psychic protective insulation that keeps a whole spectrum of energies from entering our subtle bodies, energies which would quite possibly devastate our physical and psychological health if they flowed unchecked. There is a very real danger in becoming a radionic practitioner. I have watched my radionic colleagues over the years, and have seen a number of them sicken and some die from their exposure to energies they simply did not understand. I have watched my own reactions to the field of energy that comprises a practice, so I am aware of the pitfalls and the dangers inherent in this work. This danger is magnified and augmented by the very act of making a radionic diagnosis, something every practitioner does day in and day out. During diagnostic work one is directly exposed to the pathological imbalances of the patient, these can leech into the practitioner's own subtle bodies unless he or she knows how to keep them out. To this we can add the often destructive power of self-transformation; let me explain. When radionic diagnosis is made the supersensory faculties of the practitioner are brought into play, constant practice opens up areas of the psyche and unless the practitioner consciously controls this ongoing and enhanced process of transformation, sooner or later the energies contacted and utilised in the work will run into resistance, and resistance if persisted in may eventuate in the ultimate transformation of death, or at the very least a series of inner crisis points.

Radionic practitioners are of course not alone in this process but the psychic nature of their work does heighten the negative effects. Consider how high the rate of drug abuse and alcoholism is amongst medical doctors, and the suicide rate of psychiatrists. They too soak up the negative energies from their patients – just imagine listening all day to descriptions of pathological states, especially those of an astral emotional nature issuing from one neurotic or psychotic patient after another. At the end of the day the practitioner is saturated and surrounded by a soup of pathological energies, which will literally permeate and taint the very substance of his own etheric and astral bodies, especially the latter. In my previous book *Radionics: Science or Magic?* I put forward the theory that radionics was more akin to magic than science, and this is a fact – practitioners need to recognise this in order to fully understand the dangers they are exposing themselves to. To work in radionics is to handle energies in a creative and therefore magical way. In *A Treatise on White Magic* Alice Bailey points out that the magician who creates thought-forms must learn to stand at the midway point between land and water, land and water being metaphors for the mental and astral planes, and care must be taken lest the waters of the astral plane overwhelm the magician. The same applies to any radionic practitioner, they must learn to stand at the point of balance. What then does this involve in practical terms?

Firstly we must understand that any practitioner who is focused in his or her astral body and works through the solar plexus chakra is heading for trouble. Remember that 95% of all disease originates on the astral and etheric levels, and to be focused on those levels means exposure to many destructive energies especially when doing diagnostic work or treating at a distance. It is essential to disassociate the astral and etheric auras from the field of work and to be focused in the head chakras and on the mental plane at the higher levels. Empathy and identification with a patient's disease indicates a state of astral focus and will inevitably lead to trouble which will make itself felt in fatigue and an acutely oversensitive nervous system. Polarisation on the mental plane is the only safe barrier; to this must be added the capacity to work with the energy of Love through the heart chakra, in fact the head and heart chakras must be linked and working in unison for full protection. So you see, while adding the subtle dimension of chakra and subtle body diagnosis to radionics greatly increased its scope, it also set up a situation in which practitioners would be obliged to practice in a more aware state. In other words sooner or later they would be forced to acknowledge the danger inherent in the radionic process, and seek the means to overcome the destructive energies that their daily work brought them into contact with. What I am saying of course applies to all forms of healing work, but it is particularly true of radionics.

The practice of radionics forces psychic and ultimately spiritual growth, especially when it involves the practitioner in the afore-mentioned areas of diagnosis related to chakras and subtle body states. One cannot venture into such areas without due preparation and the constant vigilance required of the true healer. Later on in the book I will deal with just what this type of vigilance involves and how to adopt a posture of aligned awareness.

For several years now I have been employing a new aspect of diagnosis in my radionic work, that of ray analysis. I touched on this in *Radionics: Science or Magic?* very briefly in order to push the concept out into the mainstream of radionics and see how practitioners reacted to the idea. The reaction has been very muted and hesitant, this of course does not surprise me because in the final analysis it takes at least three years of study to begin to even come to grips with the basic concepts that are required when using this theme of spiritual psychology in relationship to radionic analysis work. It is an area of knowledge that is not easily penetrated, and with good reason – here the practitioner is touching upon potent streams of energy which must be worked with in a careful and knowledgeable manner.

Many people find the writings of Alice Bailey difficult to come to grips with, perhaps because the vibratory quality of her work is strictly along mental lines and does not appeal to those who are astrally focused or have a ray structure which makes other approaches to the path more readily accessible. I have studied most esoteric teachings but find the Kabbala very difficult to approach, however I can read Bailey with an ease that used to surprise me. In a curious way the lives of many people who knew Alice Bailey personally have touched upon my own – Victor Fox who was her secretary for many years was a neighbour and close friend of mine in California, and there are others, most of whom have passed into the Light, who imparted much knowledge to me along the lines of A.A.B.'s writings. I suppose some twenty four years of studying Bailey's work, especially in respect to the subject of healing and spiritual psychology, have naturally led me to apply this knowledge to the field of radionics – this is after all a practical application of esoteric healing. Having a lot of theory about healing is all very well, perhaps essential, but it is the practical application that matters. By introducing the idea of chakra and subtle body diagnosis into radionics, I set a stream of energy into motion which has both broadened and deepened the practice of this remarkable healing art, and at the same time it has heightened the awareness of practitioners in respect to the subtle energy bodies which underlie the physical form. Now I want to round out this process by making a more detailed presentation of the seven rays, and showing at the same time just how this knowledge can be applied in a practical manner in radionic work. No one should be daunted by the fact that Bailey wrote five large volumes on the subject of the rays, there are certain fundamental aspects of this knowledge which can be understood and applied in practice.

Not surprisingly this area of esoteric knowledge carries its own protective boundary or ring-pass-not. The practitioner has to penetrate this body of information with a pure motive, this means that the knowledge acquired is for the use of serving others, not self-agrandisment or to bolster the image of the personality. There must be a high level of creative interest in the subject matter, and an enthusiastic search for knowledge – this approach enables the practitioner to touch upon the real knowledge of the rays which is simply not available from cursory reading. The knowledge of the rays has to be transformed to self-knowledge, it has to be absorbed so that it becomes a part of the individual. As this happens the barriers recede to give way to greater awareness, thus the practitioner renders himself effective. It is not enough to know that the First Ray has this or that quality, or that the virtues of the Second Ray are patience, endurance, love of truth and so on. These energies have to become a living reality in the consciousness of the practitioner before they can be commented upon and utilised in diagnostic work in a practical manner. In other words the practitioner is forced to expand his awareness, and this is what I have said all along, radionics is more than a healing art it is a powerful impetus to self-transformation, and unless practitioners are aware of this and aware of the nature of the energies they are handling, they court danger and possibly disaster.

While the response of radionic practitioners to my last book has been less than enthusiastic, possibly because it upset too many highly anomalous sacred cows that infest this healing art, the response from doctors and psychologists and some independent thinking practitioners has been very, very encouraging. Many said, that finally they could see what radionics was really about, and that what I had written in *Radionics: Science or Magic?* voiced what they had felt for many years. Francis Farrelly a veteran practitioner visited me in Chichester and echoed these sentiments, and said that it was about time someone cleared the air and clarified what radionics was all about, that is the esoteric constitution of man and not instrumentation, because the latter can often serve to blind the practitioner to the real importance and understanding of the human instrument and its unfoldment, and to the nature of the energies involved.

Perhaps more important than these letters, phone calls and personal comments supporting the themes pursued and outlined in *Radionics: Science or Magic?* is the fact that the book initiated a number of contacts, one of them with a psychologist in Europe who guides and teaches several groups along the lines of spiritual psychology. He wrote to me in late 1983 saying amongst other things that:

> It was a relief for me when you definitely distinguished the process of analysis and healing from the use of apparatus, as you did clearly in the last book *Radionics: Science or Magic?* (At the same time this last book is, in my opinion, the most unfinished book; it is an in-between book, I think.)

Well I would have to agree with this. The book served a number of purposes, the primary one being to establish a more up-to-date viable basis for radionics, so that it could leave the anomalies and idio-syncracies behind and develop towards its vast potential. The resistance to the concepts outlined, amongst the orthodox power structure in organised radionics was immediately apparent and still continues to manifest itself. How important this is I do not care to speculate, I only know that the unfoldment of radionics will not be halted by biased and uninformed opinion. When any organisation crystalizes it must eventually shatter and give way to the new impulse. That impulse is now beginning to flow into radionics, on one hand it brings with it divisiveness as those of the old school try desperately to hang onto their cherished ideas which have long since served their purpose. At the creative level radionics is moving into a new expression, dealing with the whole man in terms of energy – the seed is germinating which will give rise to a truly holistic healing art. My psychologist friend was right, *Radionics: Science or Magic?* was an unfinished, in-between book. I saw it as a preliminary statement which would lead the way to a clear exposition of the ray energies and how they formed the basis for the new frontier in radionics. In a sense I am encouraged by the fact that response to this expansion has come, not from the radionic community itself, so much as from the psychologists and doctors who are interested in radionics but have never become actively involved due to the obvious anomalies that have gone unchallenged until recently. This state of affairs is now changing, and the new impulse will give rise to a new form of radionic practice that will involve counselling as a primary approach to healing.

I see the time when properly trained radionic practitioners will be called upon to determine holistic energy profiles of patients for psychologists and psychiatrists, and that these will be used as a guide in counselling work in the future. The precedent for this approach has already been set – Dr Carl Jung certainly used the astrological charts of his patients to enhance his knowledge of them and thus his capacity to initiate a healing process. Over the past few months I have had the privilege of drawing up a whole series of charts for the psychologist in Europe, outlining the rays, the states of the chakras and organ systems of each patient and correlating them into a meaningful pattern which in the context of group work can serve as a basis for understanding the nature of personal crisis and equally important, personal potential.

Having said this, let us see just what is involved in this process and the responsibility it lays upon the practitioner. It is not an area that should be entered into lightly, because it requires considerable knowledge to deal with life patterns, and the practitioner must be able to work clearly at the mental level free from the illusory thrall of the astral plane. Not least of course is the very real responsibility intrinsic to this form of work.

CHAPTER TWO

THE PATTERNS OF LIFE

I would call your attention to the increasing use by psychologists and thinkers of the race of the word "pattern". It is a word which has a deep occult significance.

Esoteric Psychology II – Alice A. Bailey

The pattern that most concerns us is the pattern that lies in the various aspects of the human psyche. Over the centuries man has sought to put into language his grasp and understanding of self, and herein lies the difficulty. Language veils and hides the truth, so it is vital to recognize that what we seek to understand lies beyond these words and is in no way confined by them. Paradoxically words are living entities possessing spirit, soul and form, and can be used to open the door to deeper realms of understanding and awareness.

In this book we are going to try and come to some form of clearer understanding regarding the subtle anatomy of man, and this raises some very real problems. Bailey when describing the soul and personality as a major and lesser energies says:

I would here remind you, as I have oft done before, that words fail to express and language handicaps rather than aids the objective I have in view. Human thought is now entering a field for which there exists, as yet, no true language-form, for we have no adequate terms, and in which word–symbols mean but little.

So in a sense we begin with a real disadvantage, but a beginning must be made, so where should we start and just how much detail should be covered? Bailey wrote several thousand pages on the subject of the esoteric constitution of man, the ray energies and spiritual psychology – is it possible to extract from several million words a simple yet comprehensive pattern that will provide a basis to work from in radionic practice? Well I think it is possible, but I stress it is only a basic structure which each practitioner will have to build upon for themselves. This is an area of knowledge of extreme complexity, however this should daunt no one from proceeding along these lines, albeit with care and consideration.

We can begin by accepting the Theosophical model of man as a working hypothesis, to be utilised and tested, and if need be discarded should it prove in any way inadequate. This model posits that each human being consists of a spirit, soul and personality. The personality is comprised of the mental body, the emotional body and the etheric body. The dense physical body is seen simply as an externalisation of the subtle bodies, not a principle in itself but reflecting patterns of the inner energy structures of the subtle anatomy. When an esotericist speaks of the 'physical' body he usually means the etheric body. There is no such thing as a physical/etheric body – this term however seems to have been somewhat misunderstood in radionic circles, possibly because I used it initially to point out that the etheric body is the 'physical' body from an esoteric point of view. Perhaps it is necessary to simply speak of the etheric body as the etheric body and leave the term physical body for the dense physical form.

Each aspect of the esoteric constitution of man is qualified by a ray energy. So there is the ray of the monad or spirit, the ray of the soul, the ray of the mental body, the ray of the emotional body and those of the etheric body and personality. The personality ray comes into being when the individual has brought about a degree of integration between the various bodies of the lower-self. As we shall see later the ray of the soul and the ray of the personality provide us with certain insights as to the nature of physical and psychological disease.

These rays then form the life-pattern of the individual and confer upon him his strengths and weaknesses, his potential and limitations. In times of inner crisis an understanding of these ray energies and their effects can serve as a focal point from which a new awareness and orientation can be achieved. This of course is not done by distant treatment so much as through counselling on a group or one to one basis, or by correspondence. The former is to be preferred because there is the direct interaction between the therapist and his client which enables the energies of both to be utilised more fully.

What then are the rays? According to Bailey they are seven great streams of energy, and that every form in nature is to be found upon one ray or another. The interplay of these rays produces the myriad of forms we see in the world and indeed in the universe itself. They are looked upon as the first differentiation of the Divine Triplicity, in the Bible they are designated as the Seven Spirits before the Throne of God, and the christian mystic Jacob Boehme frequently refers to them in *Aurora* as the seven Fountain Spirits.

Of what use is knowledge of the rays to the practitioner and the patient? There are many uses, first it enables us to understand our various mental, emotional and physical tendencies. Secondly we can more clearly gauge our abilities, opportunities, limitations and capacities. With the insight knowledge of our ray makeup brings, it is possible to determine our real vocation more accurately and not least our field of service to humanity. To know our rays is to know ourselves – this is what is meant by the words – 'Man know thyself, then thou shalt know the universe and God.' This theme is repeated again and again in all esoteric teachings, in the Gnostic teachings Thomas the Contender writes:

> Whoever has not known himself has known nothing, but he who has known himself, has at the same time already achieved knowledge about the depths of all things.

This is a remarkable, sweeping statement when you stop to think about it. To know oneself is to acquire knowledge about the *depths* of *all* things. How so? Perhaps the key lies in the fact that all things are conditioned and qualified by the seven rays, and through an understanding of those rays as they manifest in us, we are given the key which unlocks the Mysteries. To know oneself is not to know one's name or one's profession, or the myriad things that we attach to ourselves to form an identity – to know oneself is to know what ray energies we are comprised of. We have to see ourselves as energy rather than form. In her book *The Rays and The Initiations* Bailey writes:

> Students should familiarise themselves with the "energy concept" and learn to regard themselves as energy units displaying certain types of energy.

In order to do this it is essential to understand the rays of each aspect of the personal and transpersonal self, and to observe their interactions which give rise to how we act and react in everyday life. The way we act and react is of course not so simple and other factors have to be taken into consideration. We must know for example where the focus of our life lies – is it in the astral body and manifesting through the solar plexus chakra, or is it on the mental level and working through the throat, head and heart chakras? It may in fact be some of each, although there is generally a definite primary focus of astral or mental orientation. We must also have some knowledge of the states of our chakras and just how active or underactive they are, because their effects upon the endocrine system will in no small measure dictate the state of our physical and psychological fitness.

One way of arriving at such knowledge is through radionics which employs the supersensory aspect of touch. With the right training and sensitivity it is possible to determine the ray makeup of an individual, and the states of the chakras as well as the functional integrity of the organ systems at an etheric level. This data or life-pattern can then be correlated to form a holistic picture of the patient and used in discourse on a one to one basis to aid them through whatever crisis they may be passing through at the time. This data is like a mirror, to be held up for the patient so that they can observe their own reflection, and this is important because the reflection will carry not only the limitations that they now perceive, but also their deeper potential and abilities.

In *Radionics: Science or Magic?* I devised the following schema to illustrate the subtle bodies of man and their ray energies.

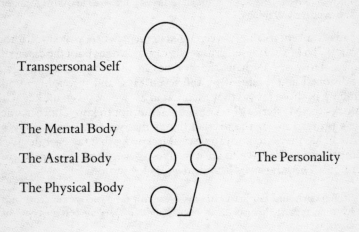

In that book I deliberately restricted my presentation of ray material because I wanted it to serve as an introduction. The two or more pages involved were more in the nature of a pebble thrown into the radionic pond to see what ripples would be created on its surface. There have been several very interesting reactions that I will not comment on here, suffice to say that time will prove the importance of this aspect of radionics, and the need for a thorough grounding in the subject before adding it to analysis work. Already there are those who have leapt in where the proverbial angels fear to tread. It is my hope that this book will prove to be both cautionary and encouraging, for I have no doubt that radionics stands on the brink of a new expansion, but to inaugurate it properly will require a particular quality and depth of knowledge with regard to the seven rays.

You may have noted that despite the fact that the monad or spirit also has a ray, I have not included it on the diagram. While we may keep in mind that the monad does of course have a ray it is of no vital import to our work in radionics. The monad is always on the 1st, 2nd or 3rd ray.

The transpersonal self, the personality and any one of its components will be found on all rays, and as a rule these change from lifetime to lifetime in order that the indwelling man learn to master their various qualities, rendering the glamours and vices inoperable and expressing the virtues.

Before going into any detail as to how these rays operate through the individual it will be necessary to outline some pertinent information about each of the rays, then we can proceed to see how their effects bring about harmony or a lack of it in the energy unit known as man.

CHAPTER THREE

THE SEVEN GREAT BUILDERS

We may, however, expect the "science of the rays" to develop rapidly in the coming era, for it promises much new understanding of human nature and behaviour.

The Seven Rays of Energy – Michal Eastcott

The seven rays or builders offer any one individual the scope for a lifetime's study, more in fact. It is as I have already mentioned a highly complex subject, and I run the risk of misleading you if I simplify it too much. However if I can outline the basic information on this fascinating subject, and indicate just how it can be employed in a radionic practice, then this book will have served its purpose.

There are seven rays, but it is important to realise that the seven rays that are our concern are the sub-rays of the 2nd ray. We live in a 2nd ray system, a system in which Love and Wisdom are being developed and expressed. Christ and the Buddha are the main exponents of this ray. Having understood that the seven rays are in fact the sub-rays of the 2nd ray we can allow this fact to recede and just think of the seven rays. I will list them in the customary manner, and then provide further details about each one.

The Rays of Aspect. These partake of the Father's Nature.
1st Ray.   Power, Will and Purpose.
2nd Ray.   Love-Wisdom.
3rd Ray.   Active Intelligence.

The Rays of Attribute. These partake of the Mother's Nature.
4th Ray.   Harmony through Conflict.
5th Ray.   Science or Knowledge.
6th Ray.   Idealism or Devotion.
7th Ray.   Order or Ceremonial Magic.

Each ray has a colour attributed to it, and these I list below along with the ray-chakra relationship.

1st Ray   Red   Crown chakra
2nd Ray   Blue   Heart chakra

3rd Ray	Yellow	Throat chakra
4th Ray	Orange	Brow chakra
5th Ray	Green	Sacral chakra
6th Ray	Violet	Solar Plexus chakra
7th Ray	Indigo	Base chakra

Having listed these colour relationships it is important to know that they deal with one viewpoint. Rays have an esoteric colour and an exoteric colour, so I will list these as well, and add one or two other correlations that might prove useful. You will note that this list is not the same as the above, this is one of the paradoxes that begins to emerge at a certain level of consciousness in which contradictory statements may be both correct or even incorrect if the writer is employing a blind to keep information from the uninitiated. Both Madame Blavatsky and Alice Bailey employed blinds particularly in respect to colour, so keep an open mind.

Rays	Exoteric Colour	Esoteric Colour	Bodily Location
1st	Orange	Red	Vital airs in skull
2nd	Indigo with a Purple tinge	Light blue	The heart
3rd	Black	Green	Centres up spine
4th	Cream	Yellow	None listed
5th	Yellow	Indigo	Brain
6th	Red	Silvery Rose	None listed
7th	White	Violet	None listed

I have not included this list for any other reason than to illustrate the need to keep an open mind on the subject. On the subject of colours and chakras one finds an often bewildering list of specific colours attributed to certain chakras. Like the ray colour correlations they frequently appear to contradict each other, but we shall take a further look into this when I deal with the chakras later in the book.

Let us take a look now at each ray and its qualities. I will endeavour to draw this material together in a form that will prove to be of practical use, so that it can be referred to when drawing up reports or when counselling a patient.

THE FIRST RAY. THE RAY OF WILL OR POWER.

This is the energy of will and power than can work out as the

destroyer of form, it unleashes the destruction that produces liberation.
Some of its esoteric titles are as follows:

> The Lord of Death
> The Liberator from Form
> The Most High
> The Will that breaks into the Garden
> The Lord of the Burning Ground

It confers a purposeful attitude, natural leadership qualities, a great
deal of positive drive. A directness in personal relationships and the
carrying out of tasks, and the ability to initiate activities and to govern
men. Where this ray is really active you will have the person with a real
sense of destiny and an innate sense of power. They are almost always
convinced that their ideas and attitudes are right. They certainly do not
suffer fools gladly, they are self-reliant and courageous. This is the ray
of the soldier, ruler, statesman, explorer and leader. Its higher expression
expresses itself through the science of statesmanship and government.
The lower expression is through modern diplomacy and politics.

First ray people (if one can use such a phrase) are inclined to be
ambitious and arrogant with a love of power, they often lack consideration for others and are prone to impatience and irritability. There
is a tendency in them to be inflexible and to resist change. Michal
Eastcott points out that history is rich with 1st ray types and lists the
following examples: Roosevelt, Churchill, Napoleon, Genghis Khan,
Alexander the Great, Hitler and Mussolini. Bailey adds Walt Witman,
Luther, Carlyle and Lord Kitchener.

Each ray has its virtues, vices and glamours. Virtues and vices are
straightforward enough but glamours are the insidious, illusory
qualities of a ray which can deflect us from the truth – glamours are like
a mist that veils and distorts reality – glamours are most likely to plague
us in everyday life without us fully recognising their presence.

Special Virtues:
Strength, courage, steadfastness, truthfulness arising from absolute
fearlessness, power to rule, capacity to grasp great questions and
concepts in a large minded way, and to handle men and measures.

Vices:
Pride, ambition, wilfulness, hardness, arrogance, desire to control
others, anger and obstinacy.

Glamours:
Love of power and authority. Pride and selfish ambition. Impatience
and irritation, separativeness, coldness, aloofness and self-centred.

Virtues to be acquired:
Tenderness, sympathy, humility, tolerance, patience. A sense of caring for others.

THE SECOND RAY. THE RAY OF LOVE-WISDOM.

This is the ray of universal love, intuition, insight, co-operation, philanthropy and wisdom. Upon this stream of energy emerge the sages, teachers, healers and reformers of humanity, their quest according to Geoffrey Hodson is to heal, teach, serve, illumine and to save their fellow men. The higher expression of teaching along this line of energy lies the initiatory processes of the Illumined Ones. The lower expression through religion.

The nature of the 2nd ray is inclusiveness and magetism. The person on this ray is inclined to be naturally sympathetic with a genuine concern for others, they are usually well-liked and mix easily. they are the peace makers but have a strong tendency towards negativity. They are easily deflected from their purpose or their views change with the company they keep. Their weaknesses are sentimentality, sensuality and a tendency to be impractical at times. The 2nd ray person is as a rule highly sensitive, sometimes too much so for their own good. Their sharp perception endows them with a facility for seeing beyond surface events and they are easily able to comprehend the subjective nature of circumstances and events. They are almost always ready to help others and frequently find their way into the helping and healing professions. Michal Eastcott lists Mother Teresa of Calcutta and Pope John Paul II as being on the 2nd ray.

Special Virtues:
Calm, strength, patience and endurance, love of truth, faithfulness, intuition, a serene temper and a clear intelligence.

Vices:
Coldness if the wisdom aspect is overemphasized, indifference to others, contempt of mental limitations in others, over absorption in studies.

Glamours:
Fear. Negativity. A poor self-image. A sense of inferiority and inadequacy. Depression, constant anxiety, self-pity. Excessive self-effacement, inertia and ineffectiveness.

Virtues to be acquired:
Love, compassion and unselfishness.

People on this ray are rarely satisfied with what they have attained in life, they never feel that they have really accomplished anything, even when their accomplishments are very obvious to others. Fear and anxiety are very real burdens to these people due to their innate sensitivity. The 2nd ray healer according to Bailey works best by thoroughly knowing the temperament of the patient and the nature of the disease so as to use his or her will power to the best advantage.

The 2nd ray energy is sometimes referred to as:

> The Displayer of Glory
> The Radiance in the Form
> The Great Geometrician
> The Cosmic Christ
> The Lord of Eternal Love

While these names may seem like some sort of peculiar title, the truth is that they are potent seed-thoughts for any healer to meditate upon. This of course applies to all of the names of the ray Lords.

THE THIRD RAY. THE RAY OF ACTIVE INTELLIGENCE.

This is the ray of creative ideation, adaptability, impartiality, dignity, comprehension and understanding. It is also the ray of industry, business, technology (witness the present computer boom), communications and transport. This is the ray that has brought man from the caves of prehistoric times to our present state of technical ability. People on this ray are usually successful in business and can handle money efficiently and wisely. They have an ability to plan things out and instinctively know the most economic way to achieve their ends. They are often physically well co-ordinated – jogging is a 3rd ray pastime as are all athletic endeavours. The 3rd ray is the power that evokes the form, it is the ray of the true builder. It has the power to evolve, the quality of mental illumination and the ability to produce synthesis on the physical plane. Individuals who speak quickly and make rapid movements often have a 3rd ray physical body. They may chatter incessantly about little or nothing, and like to appear busy at all times with no time to spare.

Some of the names applied to this ray are:

> The Builder of the Foundation
> The Great Architect of the Universe
> The Dispenser of Time
> The Lord of Memory
> The Illuminator of the Lotus

According to Hodson this is the ray of the astrologer, scholar, diplomat, philosopher, judge, banker, economist, chess player, strategist and director. These professions that are allied to the rays will serve as a guide when discussing such matters with your patients. I frequently have radionic patients who say to me that they are in a time of crisis and transition in their life and they are looking to change direction and move along a new tack. By using the ray guides it is possible to discuss which lines of direction might prove the most useful.

The higher method of teaching truth along the 3rd ray stream of energy is through all means of communication and interaction. Radio, telegraph, television, telephone and transportation. The lower expression is through the use of spread of money and gold. The 3rd ray type can be something of a manipulator and we see this in the way the Gnomes of Zurich play with the gold and money markets to serve their own ends. Political scheming and working in devious ways are both 3rd ray expressions of energy.

Special Virtues:
Wide views on all abstract questions, sincerity of purpose, a clear intellect, capacity for concentration on philosophic studies, patience, caution and an absence of the tendency to worry himself or other people over small trifling matters.

Vices:
Intellectual pride, coldness, isolation, inaccuracy in details, absent-mindedness, obstinacy, selfishness, over-critical of others.

Glamours:
The glamour of always being busy. Materialism. Preoccupation with detail which may paralyse action because so many angles to a situation are evident. Efficiency and self-importance through being the one who knows. Scheming and manipulation of others. Deviousness and self-interest.

Virtues to be acquired:
Tolerance, devotion, common sense, accuracy and sympathy.

The healer on this ray works best by using drugs made of herbs or minerals belonging to the same ray as the patient. This is something I will deal with in more detail in a later chapter. Clearly this is the ray of the herbalist and the homoeopathic physician – and just imagine how their capacity to heal would be improved if they knew the rays of the patient and the remedies available to them.

THE FOURTH RAY. THE RAY OF HARMONY THROUGH CONFLICT

This is often spoken of as the ray of the artist, the mediator and the interpreter. This ray confers an inherent sensitivity to colour and form in right proportion, and a capacity to create artistically. These people often have excellent gifts but the inertia aspects of this ray may prevent them from really expressing them fully. This leads to frustration and discontent and the creative potential may be lost due to depression and despondency. There is a tendency towards ambivalence, vacillation and instability. There is also a strong drive towards dissipating energies through too many avenues at one time. 4th ray people are often impulsive and over-react to stressful situations. They can be hyperactive one moment and indolent another. While conflict marks this ray, harmony is its primary role – the 4th ray mediator can bring harmony into situations of conflict. Sometimes if life appears a little dull the 4th ray person will stir up conflict in their environment just to feel alive.

Some of the names of this ray energy are:

> The Perceiver on the Way
> The Divine Intermediary
> The Corrector of the Form
> The Dweller in the Holy Place

Special Virtues:
Strong affection, sympathy, physical courage, generosity, devotion, quickness of intellect and perception.
Vices:
Self-centredness, worrying, inaccuracy, lack of moral courage, strong passions, indolence and extravagance.
Glamours:
Diffusion of interests and energy. Impracticality and the glamour of imagination, grandiose schemes. Vagueness and a lack of objectivity. Constant inner and outer conflict, causing argument and acrimony. Dissatisfaction because of sensitive response to that which is higher, better and more beautiful.
Virtues to be acquired:
Serenity, confidence, self-control, purity, accuracy, mental and moral balance, unselfishness.

The approach to healing is through massage and magnetism. The higher mode of teaching truth is through the deeper aspects of Masonic work. The lower expression is through modern city planning and architectural construction.

Bailey points out that this is the ray of combat and struggle. This leads to the "Birth of Horus" or the Christ within. These people know the frustration of not being able to express the perfection they can sense. They are often in a state of stress and their conversation can range from brilliant to non-existent as they lapse into long gloomy silences. Their quest and driving impulse is to harmonise and beautify.

THE FIFTH RAY. THE RAY OF CONCRETE KNOWLEDGE AND SCIENCE

This is the ray of the lower mind which has influenced education and given rise to science. It is the ray of the lawyer, scientist, mathematician, physicist and astronomer. People on this ray analyse and quantify, they won't tolerate woolly thinking and need to see everything measured and proven according to orthodox standards. They are not into subjective spiritual realities that cannot be clearly defined in their terms. Like the 3rd ray type they are critical and tend to be separative in their attitudes. They like mental gymnastics and the opportunity to flex their discriminatory muscles. 5th ray medicine has no time for any other approaches to healing, they are all below its 'imagined' high level of excellence. Narrow convictions, intellectual pride and prejudice, intense materialism as expressed in the use of crude and destructive drugs are all a part of this ray. I should add however, so are all of the excellent benefits that science has brought us. Bailey states that it will be the scientist who leads the way into the esoteric realms, not the theologian or mystic. Today the new physics is witness to the truth of her statement made in the 1930's.

Some of the names given to this ray have a clear connection with some of the above listed qualities.

> The Revealer of Truth
> The Dispenser of Knowledge
> The Dividing Sword
> The Guardian of the Door

Special Virtues:
Perseverance, common sense, justice without mercy, strictly accurate statements, uprightness, independence, keen intellect. Perceptive mental penetration and application.
Vices:
Narrowness, lack of sympathy, an unforgiving temper, harsh criticism, prejudice, little reverence.
Glamours:
Constant analysis and splitting of hairs, criticism, overemphasis of form while neglecting the life aspect, cold mental assessment and disparagement of feeling, intellectual pride, reason, proof and intellectuality are sacrosanct.
Virtues to be acquired:
Reverence, devotion, sympathy, love and wide-mindedness.

The 5th ray person approaches healing through surgery and electricity, the modalities of physiotherapy.

Punctuality and orderliness are 5th ray qualities and the person on this ray will teach through the use of diagrams, detailed explanations and charts. The higher approach to teaching truth is through the science of the soul, that is esoteric psychology. The lower is through the modern educational system.

The 5th ray drives people to discover and they have a strong thirst for knowledge. They achieve through seeking, searching, probing, patient observation and experimentation. Their ability to put their feelings behind them and their thirst for knowledge, leaves no doubt in their minds that laboratory experiments on animals are justifiable. A 2nd ray person on the other hand finds such experimentation horrifying. 5th ray people hate to be proved wrong or to admit mental defeat.

THE SIXTH RAY. THE RAY OF DEVOTION.

This ray is the energy that fuels idealism and nationalistic attitudes. Religious wars and crusades all originate on this energy, it is clearly quite active in the world at this time but began to pass out of this cycle of manifestation according to Bailey in 1625 A.D. We are presently seeing its final and more destructive throes. It is the ray of the saint, mystic, martyr and evangelist. The person in this ray is full of religious instincts and it involves intense personal feelings, religious instincts and impulses. The Inquisition was a manifestation of 6th ray energy, and those carrying it out felt it quite in order to burn people at the stake in order to 'save' their souls. To the 6th ray person everything is either perfect or intolerable, they must have a personal god and are often bigoted and fanatical. Blind devotion to personalities be they a political killer or spiritual guru is an expression of the 6th ray. The deprecate, ignore or despise the intellect. Their loyalty to a cause, good or bad will be strong and they will work with one-pointedness, ardour and a fiery enthusiasm for what they believe in. Bailey states that the 6th ray has set its mark upon humanity more than any other ray, and points out that it has produced the corrupt and awful story of man's cruelty to man.

Some of the names given to this ray are:

> The Divine Robber
> The Crucifier and the Crucified
> The Devotee of Life
> The Hater of Forms
> The Warrior on the March

Special Virtues:
Devotion, single-mindedness, love, tenderness, intuition, loyalty and reverence.

Vices:
Partiality, over-dependence on others, selfish and jealous love, self-deception, prejudice, sectarianism, fiery anger and over rapid conclusions.

Glamours:
Fanaticism, narrow mindedness, love of the past and existing forms, possessiveness and exaggerated devotion, reluctance to change, rigidity and too much intensity of feeling. Hero worship.

The Virtues to be acquired:
Strength, purity, self-sacrifice, truth, tolerance, serenity, balance, common sense and flexibility.

The 6th ray healer works through faith and prayer and teaches through inspiration. It teaches truth in its higher expression through Christianity and diversified religions. The lower expression through churches and religious organisations. Michal Eastcott points out that the high idealism surrounding King Arthur and his Knights of the Round Table and the Grail Legends, with their altruism and high ideals of chivalry are 6th ray expressions. There seems to be two types of 6th ray people, those who are visionaries and militant leaders and those who are the devotional servers. One type can be overbearing and filled with impetuous drives while the other is content to be rather soft and easily led.

THE SEVENTH RAY. THE RAY OF CEREMONIAL MAGIC OR ORDER.

This ray gives us the rules for law and order. It is the ray of the ceremonialist, ritualist, magician, producer and pageant-master. Shaman, high priests, court chamberlains are a product of this ray energy. The person on this ray makes the perfect nurse or sculptor, and they are born organisers. It is the ray which functions through organisation and synthesis, and is directly related to ceremony, sex, money and government. The ordered actions of our day are a reflection of the 7th ray energy, the routine of getting up in the morning, going to the bathroom, dressing, eating breakfast and going to work are a form of ritual. In a healing practice we follow routines and procedures, case history taking, examination and consultation are all 7th ray expessions. Radionics is certainly a 7th ray healing technique very much allied to ceremonial and ritual white magic, and to the life-force which sustains man through the chakras, most notably the base chakra which it governs. 7th ray people do not like loss of outer power, humiliation, discourtesy, rudeness, frustration and adverse criticism coming from one of lesser standing. They pay great attention to detail and as a rule like pomp and ceremony. Grace, precision and ordered beauty are their thing, and they look for skill and dignity in their work and bearing.

In listing some of the names of this ray Bailey points out that they indicate the work of the future.

> The Unveiled Magician
> The Worker in the Magical Art
> The Keeper of the Magical Word
> The Divine Alchemical Worker
> The Orienting Force
> The Key to the Mystery
> The One who lifts to Life

While the 6th ray has been rapidly going out of manifestation since 1625 A.D. the 7th ray has been coming into manifestation since 1675. The teacher on this ray teaches through dramatisation and sacred language. It teaches truth in the higher expression through all forms of white magic, and in the lower expression through spiritualism.

Predictably as the 7th ray influence is felt more strongly we shall see the rise of radionics as a healing art. We have seen already a world wide interest in shamanism, witness the popularity of the books of Carlos Castaneda outlining the teachings of Don Juan, a Yaqui sorcerer. Look on the shelves of bookshops and you will see an increasing number of books on magic and shamanism, some excellent and a lot of them filled with rubbish. There will be an upsurge of interest in things magical, no doubt their will be a proliferation of workshops on how to become an urban shaman in one weekend, and while these may energise the astral bodies of the participants they will doubtless do little to awaken their higher minds to the highly creative potential of white magic.

Special Virtues:
Strength, perseverance, courage, courtesy, extreme care in details, self–reliance.

Vices:
Formalism, bigotry, pride, narrowness, superficial judgements, self–opinion over indulged. Fussiness, over–fastidiousness and given to excessive organisation.

Glamours:
Rigid adherence to law and order, over–emphasis of organisation and form, love of the secret and the mysterious, psychism, the glamour of ritual and ceremonial, a deep interest in omens and superstition.

Virtues to be acquired:
Realisation of unity, wide–mindedness, tolerance, humility, gentleness and love.

The 7th ray approach to healing is through the precise carrying out of 'orthodox' methods. The one dose, one remedy approach in homoeopathy is purist and strictly 7th ray, this is why there has been an upsurge of interest in this area of healing, but I shall say more about that later.

This material then should form for you a point of reference when interpreting the rays of a patient. It provides the basic qualities of the rays and from this can be garnered a deeper understanding which can only come through prolonged study and contemplation of these energies. They are like symbols which have to be absorbed slowly into the psyche so that the reality of these energies can come alive and be of practical use.

It is a useful exercise, in fact an essential one if you are to come to grips with this material, to draw up your own chart listing the rays you think qualify each of your bodies. It is best to do this by observing your attitudes, and listing and taking note of your reactions to everyday situations. Don't dowse out your rays, but acquire this self-knowledge through observation, heed the Delphic injunction to know yourself.

CHAPTER FOUR

RADIONIC ANALYSIS OF THE RAYS

The power of correctly registered impression, the ability rightly to interpret it and then to draw from it correct deduction, is the secret of all diagnosis where psychology is concerned.

DINA Vol. II – Alice Bailey

The above quotation sums it all up for the radionic practitioner – *correctly registered impression,* the *ability to make the right interpretation,* and then *to be able to make the correct deduction* in respect to the findings. This is not too difficult a task when dealing with the organ systems, it becomes more difficult when determining and analysing the states of the chakras, and have no illusions about ray interpretation – it is a complex matter. However a start has to be made somewhere, techniques have to be devised and utilised in practice to see how effective they are. Where they fall short of the task at hand they should be modified or discarded if necessary, and new approaches sought. This in a very real sense is pioneering work, there are bound to be mistakes made through lack of knowledge and insufficient understanding. But provided the practitioner's motives are pure and a sense of proportion is maintained then progress will ensue.

It is perhaps worth recording how and why I began to use ray analysis in my radionic practice. In the early summer of 1981 I was reviewing the changes that had taken place in radionics since the advent of my first book *Radionics and the Subtle Anatomy of Man* which was published in 1972. The chakras and subtle bodies had been introduced into radionics through this book, and practitioners had taken to these concepts and procedures quite readily. I began to reflect on the completeness of this approach, and it became more than evident that there was one more piece to be added to the pattern that would complete radionic procedure and make it the only truly holistic form of diagnosis and treatment available today.

The missing piece was ray analysis, but how would one go about utilising it? The answer came in the form of a request for a radionic analysis from a friend who was a student of Alice Bailey's writings and who also served as a secretary within the Arcane School teaching system. He had a chronic right sacro–iliac problem which nothing had been able to help effectively. I made a full analysis of the organ systems and chakras and then on a sudden inspiration I thought to myself, I'll surprise him with more data than he bargained for, so I drew up the diagram I now use for this purpose and proceeded to determine his rays through radionics. His response was one of complete surprise bordering on amazement, and he confirmed that in his opinion my analysis of his rays was virtually spot on. This feedback from someone who was well versed in Bailey's work and had spent time figuring out his own rays, encouraged me to proceed along the lines I had initiated. That was in July 1981, since then I have done several hundred such organ–chakra–ray profiles, many of them for people who are very familiar with the terminology and who have spent much time in self–observation determining their own rays, and the feedback from them is extremely positive. Even from people who are not familiar with the ray terminology I have had many responses saying that my report and interpretation of their physical well–being, the way they expressed or failed to express themselves, and their characteristics was spot on, one patient wrote – '. . . it is as though you have known me all of my life.' Such responses are very common, but what is more important, the patient has been given an insight into themselves that may or may not have been otherwise available to them.

As a rule this type of information is of use to those patients who are consciously following the spiritual path, to those who are passing through a crisis point in their lives, or who really need the insight to re–orient themselves or alter their life–style to include the call of the inner way. It is a fact that many people become ill through resisting this inner call, and practitioners, if they are to truly serve their patients must understand the signs of this resistance and be able to very carefully *hint* at the appropriate steps, which if taken might help to resolve and disperse the stress. I choose the word *hint* with care because no practitioner should assume the role of guru unless he or she wants to become immersed in the illusory patterns of glamour.

So the discriminatory faculty must be brought to bear on the matter of ray analysis – it is only suitable for certain people. If a person is suffering from an ailment and they are basically physically oriented, they could not care less about chakras or rays. As far as they are concerned they want to be well, the esoteric aspects of their disease are irrelevant, and should quite rightly remain so in most instances.

Having said all this, let us look at ways to make a ray analysis. I began by using the seven colour cards devised by Malcolm Rae as a focus or witness for each ray, but found them rather unsatisfactory. I suppose cards representing the rays could be dowsed out, but it would take someone who had been immersed in the subject for many years to arrive at a proper series of partial radii to accurately represent each ray.

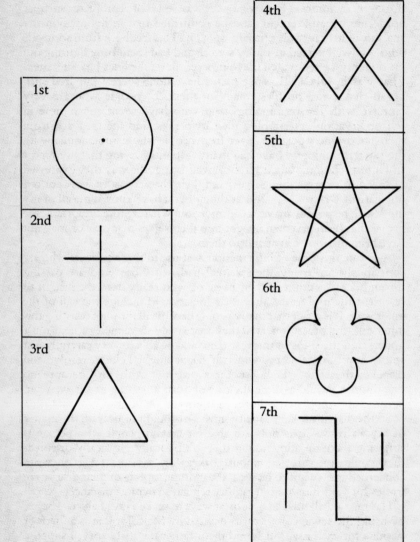

SYMBOLS REPRESENTING EACH OF THE SEVEN RAY ENERGIES.

In *Radionics: Science or Magic?* I spent some time discussing the importance of symbols in respect to the intuitive grasp of information from the Universal Mind by way of the right mind–brain hemisphere, so it was to symbols I turned in my search for an appropriate ray witness, or rather, seven ray witnesses. The following are taken from *The 7 Human Temperaments* by Geoffrey Hodson the eminent Thesophical writer and lecturer. I have found these to be quite satisfactory, and I am sure you will too. Subsequently I have devised a series of liquid homoeopathic filters which act as witnesses for the rays and these have proved excellent because of the inclusion of the appropriate ray substances or I should say, energies, in potentised form.

When dowsing out the rays of a patient it is essential to be in a composed and highly relaxed state of dynamic attention, and concentration should be unwavering. A suitable protocol for identifying the rays is as follows:

1. Place the first two fingers of your free hand on the 1st ray symbol. Swing your pendulum over the patient's witness and mentally ask if their transpersonal self is on the 1st ray.
2. Repeat this procedure until you get a positive reaction to one of the ray symbols. Then mark the number of that ray into the larger top circle of the diagram which represents the transpersonal self or soul.
3. Next repeat this process beginning with the 1st ray and working down, mentally ask is this the ray of the mental body? When you have identified it, mark the top circle of the three smaller circles which represent each of the subtle bodies.
4. The whole process is repeated for each body and finally for the personality ray.

When you have finished you should have a number in each of the circles which will provide the basis for your ray interpretation. I say basis, because there is more to the analysis. The next step, and this a most vital one, is to determine which body the transpersonal ray is predominantly working through, and which subtle body or vehicle the ray of the personality is working through. In each case these will be different bodies, and according to these findings certain capacities, characteristics and limitations will be reduced or enhanced. It is important to keep in mind that the ray analysis will provide you and the patient with a spiritual and psychological profile of themselves. Keep ever in mind that the resistance of the personality ray to the soul ray is one of the most fruitful sources of physical and psychological ill health. The battle between these ray energies is a protracted one and is fully illustrated in the Bhagavad Gita wherein Arjuna, symbol of the transpersonal self faces the ray energies of the personality on the battleground. Practitioners should find the Bhagavad Gita an interesting discourse on this process wherein the forces of the soul do battle with those of the personality. Certain ray combinations give a useful indication in some instances that the patient is in the midst of such an inner battle, and to be able to explain this to them in the appropriate terms is very therapeutic.

So our ray chart will now look something like this.

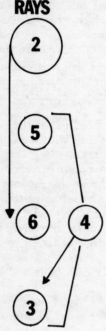

RAYS

It now clearly illustrates for us the rays of each of the various components of the higher and lower selves, and it indicates certain primary channels that have been set up by the transpersonal self before incarnation.

A word here at this point regarding incarnation and reincarnation might be in order. Despite their lack of experience in respect to ray analysis there are already 'experts' within radionics who are saying you have to subscribe to the theory of reincarnation if you are going to bring ray analysis into your practice. This of course is not so, there is no need whatsoever to have a belief in reincarnation to make use of this aspect of analysis. A profile of the organ systems, chakras and rays can be just as meaningful to a person who subscribes to the 'dead and gone' school of thought, as it can to the 'gone today and back tomorrow' brigade.

Personally I subscribe to reincarnation but there is no need to make an issue of it. I would add however that by bringing this aspect into consideration a far broader picture can be obtained. Our previous incarnation moulds to some extent our present ray makeup, and if for example we have had a tendency to isolate ourselves in a previous incarnation, living as a hermit or recluse, we are likely to bring this tendency through into the present life in the form of bodies on the line of will, that is rays 1, 3, 5 and 7 and if we persist to isolate ourselves a highly pathological psychological state will ensue until we learn that isolation is not the purpose of life.

The study of life trends as expressed by the patient's rays can be used to bring about modifications. People with too much 1st ray force need to learn how to activate the 2nd sub-ray of any given body so as to open the way in this and the next incarnation towards more loving and inclusive relationships. Then again people with too much 2nd ray energy, who soak up the energies and stresses and disease patterns from anything and anybody who comes near them, must learn to activate the will aspect. You can perhaps begin to see some of the real complexity of this subject, but also its fascinating and practical aspects. The rays are the very energy of life itself, a sort of 'connective tissue' as my psychologist colleague aptly described them, and once you begin to grasp the principles they will prove of inestimable value to both you and your patients.

As you can see, in principle, determining the rays of a patient is a simple process but one that requires a greater depth of awareness and sensitivity than may at first seem apparent. Ray analysis must be backed by knowledge otherwise it will prove to be a dangerous tool rather than a highly useful procedure. Anyone can dowse and come up with a set of rays for a patient – but the question will remain, how valid are the findings? My answer to that is – the findings can only be of use if the practitioner has steeped himself in the subject, it is not something that should be tackled and used on a whim or just to be 'up-to-date' and flowing with the trend. I have mentioned earlier, it is not safe to idly play around with energies in radionics, particularly if motives are mixed, because trouble can only be the outcome of such an approach.

CHAPTER FIVE

PRELUDE TO RAY INTERPRETATION

Occult students must increasingly think and work in terms of energy. These energies are spoken of esoterically as "having impulsive effects, magnetic appeals, and focused activities."

Esoteric Psychology Vol. II – Alice A. Bailey

While we may from time to time make the effort to think and work in terms of energy, the pull of form and its attraction is always present to distract us and present a different view of things. By making a constant effort to think and work in terms of energy a repolarising will take place within, until consciousness is predominantly focused at the subtler levels and ultimately within the protective mandala of the transpersonal self. It is in this state that all healing work becomes more effective, and the practitioner enjoys the 'circle of safety' which keeps negative flows of energy from entering his or her auric envelope.

In chapter three a series of ray qualities was outlined, drawn from various sources. These can serve as a basis but they are not enough to enable anyone to make a comprehensive interpretation. In this chapter I will list more material which will add a working synthesis to what has gone before. Knowing the rays and their qualities is one thing, knowing how they manifest and interact in man is quite another matter.

The seven rays are divided into the rays of love and the rays of will. The rays 2, 4 and 6 are along the line of love, they interact and have the capacity to work well together. The rays 1, 3, 5 and 7 are the rays of will, and they too work well together and interact with ease. Based on this understanding we will then know that a person with a 5th ray mental body and a 3rd ray physical will have the capacity to bring ideas through from the mind to the brain with ease, on the other hand if the physical body is on the 2nd ray then there might be some resistance. It does not mean of course that ideas and thoughts could not manifest because of the ray difference, but it might mean that the 5th and 3rd ray combination was capable of fast, precise thinking, capable of grasping ideas rapidly. I should add that it would also make for a person who tended to be critical of others. A 5th ray mind on the other hand, working through a 2nd ray physical brain may not be quite so precise, certainly the thought processes would be more tolerant and inclusive, and less critical. If we misinterpret the concept of resistance between the

1st and 2nd ray qualities, and see them as in opposition to each other we will have missed the point. It is a fact that a 1st ray soul would have little difficulty working through a 2nd ray mind because on the higher level these two rays work well together.

It is important to remember that when I write about 'a lot of 1st ray' or 'a lot of 2nd ray' in a person's ray makeup I am speaking in general about the rays 1, 3, 5 and 7, and 2, 4 and 6 respectively.

So let us look at a series of statements in respect to the rays which will further aid us in the work of interpretation. I will try where possible to keep them in some semblance of ray order, no doubt pushed in that direction by my own strong 7th ray.

1. A 1st ray soul or 1st ray personality creates the difficulty of "isolated independence" difficulty in co-operating and unadaptable. The 2nd ray can help offset these tendencies with its inclusiveness.
2. A lot of 1st ray can produce emotional instability.
3. 1st ray soul and 3rd ray personality (as in Catholic Church) gives a love of politics and temporal power, plus a preoccupation with commercial and financial matters.
4. 1st ray astral body can give rise to fanaticism, proud dependence on self-gained knowledge, surety of opinion. Imposition of ideas and judgement on others, plus a conviction that his methods are superior.
5. 1st ray can give a strong conviction of destiny, a sense of power and the feeling you can see through people from a superior position so that their faults and failures loom large in your consciousness.
6. As previously mentioned, but worth repeating, 1st and 2nd rays work well on the higher levels of consciousness.
7. 1st ray soul for forcing issues and determining results.
8. A 1st ray soul can easily impress a 1st ray brain, making the individual intuitive though not psychic. It also confers good organising power.
9. Invoking the energy of a 1st ray soul can prove hazardous if there is not sufficient 2nd ray energy to modify it.
10. 1st ray souls often "stand alone" and unless they are used to directing their energy wisely its force can shatter the weakest subtle bodies of other people, particularly if it flows through a 6th ray astral body.
11. A 1st ray soul working through a 5th ray mind, a 7th ray brain and a 5th ray personality would lead to intelligent high grade work in a chosen profession, but would negate the free play of the intuitive faculty.
12. 1st ray mind often indicates the real occult student.

13. A 1st ray astral body fosters and feeds the sense of isolation and separativeness. It also fosters fear of attachment.

14. A 1st ray astral body which has a 3rd ray personality focused in it, adds to the power of glamour in these areas.

15. 1st ray can give a sense of centralisation, of uniqueness and isolation, especially if the astral body and personality are both on this ray.

16. A 1st ray mental body can offset the 6th ray tendency to pay undue attention to details of process.

17. A 1st ray mental body and a 1st ray astral body make it difficult to establish and maintain equilibrium.

18. 1st ray mental body provides a good co-operating point for a 2nd ray soul – this combination confers strength and enhances the will–to–persist and the will–to–understand.

19. 1st ray astral body with a 3rd ray physical may create a dominance of devotional will in physical plane expression.

20. A 1st ray mental body with a 1st ray personality gives:
    (a) A sense of (sometimes unrealised) separativeness.
    (b) Makes co-operation easy in theory but difficult in practice.
    (c) A tendency to criticise.
    (d) A great facility for overactivity.
    (e) Evokes a love of power and a desire for that pleasurable sensation which comes from speech which evokes acquiescence and places you "in the seat of the superior person".

21. A 1st ray personality can isolate a person in their own mind from associates.

22. A 1st ray mind impact upon a 6th ray astral body can sweep it into dramatic over–emphasized action.

23. 2nd ray can create suffering from attachment and too rapid an identification with others and their problems. Healers please note.

24. The 2nd ray is the ray of Intuitive Love.

25. A 2nd ray personality can give the patience to cover a mass of detail needed, and persistence in the face of apparent lack of success.

26. Emphasis of wisdom aspect of 2nd ray can bring hardness into close relationships.

27. 2nd ray astral body can be useful in distributing the energy of love.

28. 2nd ray astral body confers harmlessness and understanding.

29. 2nd ray mental body makes illumination the line of least resistance.

30. 2nd ray soul and 2nd ray mental body creates a lack of mental precision, and makes it almost impossible to make clear cut decisions. This statement illustrates what I said earlier, that two similar rays in the makeup can be more of a problem (opportunity!?) than dissimilar ones.

31. A 2nd ray soul and a 2nd ray mental body make for a person who is too nice, too kind and too appreciative for words.
32. A 2nd ray astral astral body can balance 1st ray tendencies of other bodies.
33. A close relationship between a 2nd ray astral body and a 3rd ray physical can cause difficulties due to their different ways of building.
34. A 2nd ray soul and a 2nd ray mental body facilitate soul contact and make it easy to respond to soul impulses.
35. 2nd ray astral body facilitates transmission of love and light to others, confers intuitive insight.
36. Two bodies on the line of the 2nd ray combined with two on the 7th make for a powerful healer along both physical and psychological lines.
37. The 2nd and the 7th are the two major healing rays.
38. A 2nd ray soul seeking contact through a 2nd ray astral body will rapidly transmute the devotional attitudes of a 6th ray personality into universal and non-critical love. It will confer a horizontal inclusiveness and a vertical one-pointedness.
39. A 2nd ray astral body can make for ease in feeling on the astral level and the influence of intuitive energies from the buddhic plane.
30. 3rd ray physical increases the activity of a critical 5th ray personality.
41. 3rd ray physical leads into the world of business and commerce.
42. 3rd ray physical gives capacity to work on physical plane and handle money.
43. 3rd ray physical inclines to too much physical plane activity, rapid movements and rapid speech.
44. 3rd ray physical gives an active intelligent grip on life and a co-ordinated physical body.
45. A 3rd ray physical body demands change and does not like quietness and stability.
46. 3rd ray physical facilitates physical discipline. Most sportsmen are on this ray, so it must confer a love of sport and competitiveness.
47. The 3rd ray is most likely the ray of the overstriver and perfectionist.
48. A 4th ray mental body can bring illumination through conflict and determination.
49. 4th ray mental body confers pliability, a sense of relationship and a rapid grasp of mental truth.
50. 4th ray mental body confers the power to harmonise, unify and comprehend.
51. The 4th ray is the ray of creative living.

52. A 4th ray mind can be used to avert conflict and express the power to harmonise.

53. A 4th ray mental body confers a love of beauty, discrimination of beautiful things, books and art objects. The ray of the antique dealer. It gives the spirit of conflict urging ever forward to fresh victories.

54. A 4th ray mind will aid in the battle for vision and inclusiveness.

55. A 4th ray personality focused in a 5th ray mind can render the individual non-magnetic and give a vertical and not a horizontal attitude to life.

56. A 4th ray personality invoking the energies of a 2nd ray soul makes a person magnetic and a focal point of inspiration and loving service to others.

57. 4th ray mental body confers an intensity to the mystical interior life.

58. A 4th ray mental body gives a love of the arts and sciences.

59. A 4th ray mental body gives understanding intelligently applied, an ordered sense of colour, proportion and harmony. It can evoke a violent reaction to that which seems incorrect and inharmonious.

60. A 4th ray mental body can make harmony through conflict the keynote of a person's life.

61. The 5th ray is the ray of Intelligent Love.

62. 5th ray mind gives an enquiring and questioning nature.

63. 5th ray personality may lead the individual to watch, argue and criticise with themselves and circumstances. It emphasizes the critical side of one's nature.

64. A 5th ray mind may give an interest in astrology and a keen drive to seek the truth.

65. A 5th ray personality with a 6th ray astral body makes it difficult to grasp large issues.

66. A 5th ray personality can stand in the way of expressing love.

67. 5th ray mental body gives a capacity to grasp facts and the contours of the occult sciences.

68. A 6th ray mental body can confer a narrow one-pointed attitude.

69. 6th ray astral body gives a one-pointed attitude to life.

70. A 6th ray astral body can give the power to sacrifice and to produce good out of seeming evil.

71. A 6th ray astral body with a 6th ray personality will magnify emotional problems.

72. Overstimulation of a 6th ray astral body results in increased irritability, criticalness and fanaticism.

73. A well balanced 6th ray astral body can express love.

74. A 6th ray astral body with a 6th ray personality can create both

problems and spiritual opportunity. Beware of the glamour.

75. A 6th ray astral body and a 6th ray personality can greatly aid in the individual's life-task if used to channel soul energy.

76. 6th ray astral body can confer intensity of aspiration and a dynamic will to drive forward.

77. A 6th ray personality with a 7th ray physical body produces an over-interest and over-emphasis of the form side of life and group expression. This leads to devotion to known forms and ultimately crystalisation and rigidity.

78. The focusing of 6th ray personality energy in a 7th ray brain can be the psychic cause of headaches.

79. A 6th ray astral body, a 6th ray personality and a 6th ray physical creates a situation fraught with much difficulty, especially if the soul is along the same stream of energy, for example 2nd ray. Such a person would be battling for stability and at the same time fighting a strong tendency towards rigidity. Is such a 6.6.6 pattern the 'mark of the beast'?

80. A 6th ray astral body gives impressionability, and a measure of narrowness.

81. A 6th ray personality with a 1st ray astral body may make an individual prone to the beautiful but deceptive thought-forms of enlightened human beings. They think that they have contacted a Master of the Wisdom personally, when it is only a thought-form.

83. A 6th ray astral body can predicate an intense adherence to a line of thought, to an idea, a group, a person, an attitude or a preconceived notion. This can be a great asset or a major hindrance to spiritual growth depending on how it is employed and for what reasons.

83. A 6th ray astral body is likely to give a strong Christian tendency. Having said that it could equally give a Moslem one as well.

84. A 7th ray physical confers organisational power.

85. 7th ray physical gives facile expression of personality purpose.

86. 7th ray physical gives a sense of relationship between spirit and matter, soul and body.

87. A 7th ray physical gives the capacity to organise and rule.

88. A 7th ray physical and a 7th ray personality confers the power to work in many ways upon the physical plane bringing together subjective reality and outer form.

89. A 7th ray personality with a 7th ray physical combined with a 4th ray mind means that the individual with such a ray combination would have to take great care not to be ensnared by the glamour of magic.

90. A 7th ray physical body can confer an interest in music, ritual and psychoanalysis.

91. The 7th ray is a major healing ray.
92. 7th ray soul and a 6th ray personality leads to quick results on the physical plane.

We have here then a list of ninety two factors which can be employed in the interpretation of a ray analysis, and you will see, that with practice you will be able to formulate a remarkably comprehensive picture of each patient in terms of energy, and in terms that will be of practical use to them in dealing with their spiritual, psychological and physical crisis points. You may appreciate by now that I have stressed the need for real knowledge of this subject before launching into it, with good reason. Even the detail I have given here is small compared to the scope of the subject matter. However, we have to start somewhere, and as long as it is upon a sound basis, the rest will come of its own accord in good time.

CHAPTER SIX

WHEELS OF FIRE

We must disabuse our minds of the idea that these centres are *physical things*. They are whirlpools of force that swirl etheric, astral and mental matter into activity of some kind.

A Treatise on Cosmic Fire – Alice Bailey

Before we can begin to consider dealing further with the subject of ray analysis and interpretation it will be necessary to look at the chakras, not only in their relationship to the rays but from a number of other angles as well.

The seven major chakras that arise along the vertical axis of the cerebro–spinal channel, are formed by streams of force flowing from the transpersonal self. This force is initially transmitted from the Monad to the soul before it is driven down through the lower planes to form the chakras and the subtle bodies. Of the seven chakras, three are actually designated as *major* because they embody and express the three aspects of the Monad which are Will, Love and Intelligence. Thus we have:

1st Ray Will or Power.	The Monad.	The Crown chakra.
2nd Ray Love – Wisdom.	The Soul.	The Heart Chakra.
3rd Ray Intelligence.	Personality.	The Throat chakra.

The other four rays, those of attribute, govern the remaining chakras.

4th Ray Harmony through Conflict	– Brow chakra.
5th Ray Science or Knowledge	– Sacral chakra.
6th Ray Idealism or Devotion	– Solar Plexus chakra.
7th Ray Order or Ceremonial Magic	– Base chakra.

Now of what use is this knowledge to us in practice? Well that becomes clearer when you realise that the governing ray of a chakra indicates the primary energy that vitalises it, thus if you have a patient with a 6th ray astral body and an overactive solar plexus chakra, then you may deduce from that type of situation a number of possibilities, for example they may exhibit strong loyalties and be rather devotional, the church could play a central role in their lives, but if not they would have strong religious tendencies and a natural gift for prayer. On the less positive side they would be driven by intense emotions, they may be very possessive, selfish and quick tempered.

If on the other hand the solar plexus chakra was underactive, we may have an indication that they are very rigid in their attitudes, reluctant to change, prejudiced and locked into patterns of behaviour that are familiar and as far as they are concerned, protective.

What I am trying to illustrate here is that the ray governing the chakra is simply *a fact in time and space* – like the sky is blue. Our concern in analysis work with the rays and chakras, is the *'clouds in the sky'*, in other words the state of imbalance in the chakra, as this will influence to some degree the psychological and physiological manifestations that arise in the individual as a result of channelling too much or too little energy through the chakra. It must be kept in mind that in our example and in all cases, there will be a multitude of other factors that have to be considered before an accurate interpretation can be drawn forth.

It should be understood that while each of the seven rays governs an individual chakra and constitutes its primary energy, the same energy in a lesser degree is distributed to the remaining chakras which considerably broadens our picture and should serve to keep us from making dogmatic statements or arriving at narrow conclusions in respect to the way the rays and chakras interact, or what the effects will be.

Before proceeding with an outline of the anatomy of a chakra, and exploring how it affects our accuracy in diagnostic work, I want to return to an earlier statement regarding the downflow of energies from the soul or transpersonal self and the formation of the chakras. In my four previous books on radionics I gradually introduced the chart of the Planes according to Theosophy. Initially I used modified charts until in *Dimensions of Radionics* the full illustration was taken from *A Treatise on Cosmic Fire* by Alice Bailey. If words can veil the truth and mislead the uninitiated, then charts which are a further concretion of spiritual truths can be even more deceptive. If you look at the chart on page 817 of *Cosmic Fire,* under the heading: THE EGOIC LOTUS AND THE CENTERS, you will see that it illustrates the flow of energies down from the Monad, through the Spiritual Triad, forming the soul on the higher mental plane. Below that you will see the lines of various energies linking the various chakras on various levels. The permanent atoms and the mental unit are also illustrated as being on various levels. There is of course no other way to give a visual description of the esoteric constitution of man, well perhaps I should modify that statement and say I have not found one during all of the hours I have spent juggling the contents of this chart against the descriptions in the complex text that accompanies it.

The chart shows the permanent atoms on the mental, astral and etheric levels, when in truth they all lie within the lotus of the soul at the base of the inner petals. Similarly it shows lines of energy going from one plane to another from one chakra to another. This can be very misleading because it gives the impression that there are chakras on the lower mental level, then another lot of chakras on the astral and yet a further set on the etheric. This of course is not the case, there is one set of chakras, formed of mental, astral and etheric matter in an homogenous whole. The chart and the way it appears to outline energy-flows seems to have led to the misconception in some quarters that these flows constitute some kind of reality that can be treated separately. If you understand the structure of a chakra and its relationship to the planes of attenuated substance you will see that while the idea may make some sense exoterically, from an esoteric point of view it has little or no foundation at all. So treating the chakras in plane-relationships contains the seeds of illusion. It is a fact that a pathological state existing on a given level must be treated from the level above – now in making this statement I may appear to be contradicting myself but I am not – we are entering that area of paradox again which makes it extremely difficult for me to formulate in words, just what I am trying to put across. Let me say this in the hope that it will be sufficient, and leave you to penetrate to the essence of what I have stated above – if you as a practitioner, in treating chakras, see them as a whole and in relationship to the whole, and carry out your work from the *Triangle of Dominion,* there will be no need to involve yourself needlessly in the complexities which can in the final analysis cloud your understanding and hone the edges from your effectiveness. Simplicity is ever the watchword.

I want now, to deal with the structure of a chakra in detail. Why? Well for many reasons, not least of these because it is impossible to make an accurate assessment of the state of a chakra without a proper understanding of its structure. When a practitioner makes an analysis of the chakras the usual procedure is to mentally ask – Is the crown chakra overactive? underactive? or normally active? These questions are each posed in turn until a response is evident through the swing of the pendulum, and of course the process is repeated over and over until each of the chakra states has been determined. The accuracy of the practitioner's findings depends on two fundamental factors which are:

1. Knowledge of all aspects of the chakras and in particular their structure.

2. The level of the practitioner's own Self-Awareness.

As a rule these two factors go hand in hand, and the latter enables the practitioner to penetrate beyond the surface perturbations of the chakras. Let us look at this in a little more detail. If you as a practitioner simply seek for the state of the chakra, asking if it is under, over, or normally active, you are going to pick up nothing but surface noise and the general static of the chakra as it responds at one level to the daily round of mental, emotional and physical life. You will then find that your chakra analysis will in all probability show each of the seven chakras as being over or underactive. If this is so then you will need to make a very strict reappraisal of your knowledge of the subject and the way in which you are working. There are exceptions, but having done hundreds upon hundreds of chakra analysis charts over the years I have only ever had six that showed more than three, possibly four major chakras that were not functioning within their normal range, and only three of these showed an imbalance in ALL chakras.

One of these is worth reporting here. It involved a male patient who was suffering from fatigue and a persistent form of infection. Despite a detailed case history he had not listed his occupation. When I analysed the chakras I was surprised to find that all seven registered as underactive. I covered this in my report to him and expressed my surprise at these findings, I also asked him to let me know what kind of work he did. It turned out that for over two decades he had worked in a Nuclear Power station. This would indicate to me, that despite all of the shielding and protective measures taken in thess power stations, there is a highly subtle form of radiation present to which workers become exposed, and it would appear that the chakras *shut down* in order to nullify the effect of the radiation. Subsequently I did analysis work for a family in New Mexico where a great similarity of chakra imbalance was evident. It turned out that they all lived near the Atomic Plant, Los Alamos and there had actually been radiation leaks, but the authorities said that this was now all cleared from the area. Clearly the chakra readings indicated that they were still being affected. I might add at this point that X-ray technicians are also prone to this kind of chakra shut-down due to exposure to rays at a level not detectable by orthodox means.

The only other instances of charts showing all of the chakras in a state of over or underactivity, were in one case where the patient was literally at death's door and had to be resuscitated twice, and another instance where the individual's physical and psychological health was virtually in a state of complete disintegration. To find all of the chakras in a state of imbalance should be the exception, certainly not the rule. If you are finding that it is commonplace for you to arrive at such readings it will help to know why, and how to correct this erroneous way of working.

Forgive this digression but I felt it best to bring in the exceptions at this point rather than later on because they do help to illustrate what is to follow. To help clarify things and to understand why inaccurate readings are arrived at, we must, as I previously stated look at the structure of the chakra.

Chakras have been variously described as vortices of force or energy, saucer-like depressions, wheels of fire and so on. However the structure is more complex than that. It becomes necessary to understand that the three-fold influence of the Monad is reflected in the chakra, thus the chakra will in effect have three qualities, levels or tiers of petals (energies) in it which whirl around the central Bindu or Primal Point. The Bindu Point will be quiescent while the outer tier of petals will be very active, the second tier will be in various stages of unfoldment, and the inner tier less active. In the process of spiritual evolution the tiers of petals become active, naturally the outer tier dealing with the physical form and activity is going to be very active, the second tier reflecting the unfoldment of the second principle or Love aspect will also be active to some extent but less than the physical, and finally the Will aspect of the inner tier is the last to unfold.

Of the seven major chakras the brow, throat, solar plexus, sacral and base are the most active, the crown and heart are the last to unfold, thus the readings on these two, if you are correctly focussed is almost always within their normal range. The rest of the chakras are more subject to over or underactivity.

STRUCTURE OF CHAKRA   Insert Diagram

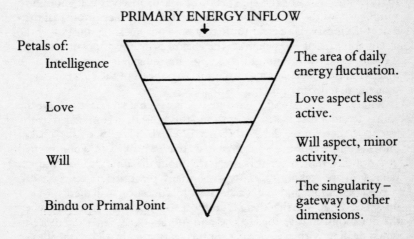

PRIMARY ENERGY INFLOW

Petals of:
  Intelligence   The area of daily
                                            energy fluctuation.

  Love   Love aspect less
                                            active.

  Will   Will aspect, minor
                                            activity.

                                            The singularity –
  Bindu or Primal Point   gateway to other
                                            dimensions.

What then are you tuning into when you seek to determine the state of a chakra? It isn't enough to mentally ask for an indication of *over* or *under* or *normal* activity, your question has to consciously encompass the three tiers of petals or energy qualities. You can forget about the Bindu Point because your consciousness could not touch upon its vibratory rate in any event. Further, unless your own chakras that you are working through are not in themselves active at the Love and Will levels to any great extent, you are only going to pick up the surface activity of the chakra anyway. I hope I am making this clear, what I am attempting to illustrate and point out is that the capacity to penetrate and touch upon the activity of the chakra is dependent upon the state of unfoldment of your own chakras and your knowledge of the structure of the chakra. This ability to penetrate the chakra is reflected in the apparently contradictory colours that are ascribed by various schools of philosophical thought. One may describe the brow chakra as being green, another red with tinges of yellow, yet another will say black – often as many as eight or nine colours will be correlated with any one chakra. Well, who is right? They all are, because as the various subtle nuances of the energy patterns of the chakra are reached through concentration, they show up as various colours all of which are valid and correct.

The lesson for us here as radionic practitioners is that anyone who analyses the states of the chakras must ask themselves is it enough to simply ask for the *over* or *under* or *normal* state, or is there more to it than that? Obviously there is far more to it, and our question must carry the ir tent and capacity to penetrate the chakra as deeply as possible so that we can obtain a meaningful reading, anything less and all you will register are the fluctuations of the surface aspects of the chakra activity which will tell you nothing of real value.

What can be done to get accurate readings? First you have to have the ability to enter the chakra in depth and this must be accompanied by the intent to determine the FUNDAMENTAL STATE of the chakra under consideration. You may use that wording in your mental question but remember it is useless without the ability to touch upon what you are seeking to know. Too many practitioners think that to wave a pendulum and to get an answer to a question is all there is to it. I hope I have showed that there is far more to it than that, especially when the questions involve the chakras and subtle bodies, and even more so when dealing with ray energies. Some years ago I broached the idea of the FUNDAMENTAL STATE of the chakra with a leading instructor in radionics – who hadn't a clue what I was talking about; which leads me to wonder just how many practitioners are actually getting factual readings in respect to their chakra analysis work. Let me repeat, if your chakra analysis charts frequently show a high proportion of the chakras out of balance, then you need to review what you are doing and then revise your approach.

This matter of levels of energy in chakras and their activity leads many people astray. I have lost track of the number of people who tell me or who claim to have had a 'kundalini' experience whatever that may be. When the kundalini energy residing in the base chakra rises up the spine with all of its force, it activates totally, not only the three tiers of petals but the bindu point as well, thus bringing about the complete transformation of the lower man into a perfected being. What many people mistakenly identify as a 'kundalini' experience is nothing more than a rising up of peripheral energies from the lower to the higher chakras up the spine which is nothing but a mere ripple compared to the real event. None of those who I have met expressed the perfection one would expect to result from the real experience, and the fact is, had it been the real thing they would never have felt the need to discuss it in the first place.

Having got onto the subject of transference of energies in rather an oblique manner, we can stay with it for a moment because the major transferences of energy from the lower to the higher chakras is a prime source of physical and psychological distress.

Bailey says of this:

The life of these three elementals is founded primarily in the three lowest centre in the etheric body:
1. The sacral centre .... the mental elemental life.
   Transferred later to the throat centre.
2. The solar plexus centre .... the astral elemental life.
   Transferred later to the heart centre.
3. The base centre .... the physical elemental life.
   Transferred later to the crown centre.

I have dealt with this elsewhere in my books on radionics, not in any great detail because it is a highly complex subject, however it is an area of knowledge that practitioners would find useful to study, because when any major transfer takes place it can bring disturbing effects in its wake, some of these may be modified through the appropriate treatment if the practitioner understands just what is involved.

Let us look at one or two factors. When the sacral energy is raised to the solar plexus which is the clearing house for all of the energies below the diaphragm, it will give rise to disturbances of the intestinal tract. When the energies of the lesser centres move to the solar plexus chakra, diseases of the gall bladder and kidneys may eventuate. Transference of energies always results in an abnormal flux and mutation of forces.

As energies gather in a chakra prior to transformation they create inflammatory states.

Bailey makes an interesting comment with respect to energy transference. She writes:

> As the heart centres and higher centres assume control, such diseases as cancer, tuberculosis and the various syphilitic complaints (due to the age old activity of the sacral centre) will gradually die out.

Energy transfer from the lower centres to the throat, will, if not utilised properly, bring about diseases of the respiratory tract and thyroid gland. This list could be extended but it is just a matter of common sense based on an understanding of energy transfer, which will provide the key to accurate diagnosis of these states. I would also direct the reader to *Esoteric Psychology Vol. II* for full details of these processes and their effects.

I hope that this chapter has served to clear up some points regarding proper analysis of the chakras and just what it involves. I have not touched upon this subject in previous books because I had mistakenly assumed that practitioners were fully cognisant of these factors, subsequently I have found this to be far from the case as witnessed by analysis sheets with all of the chakras showing marked imbalances. Common sense should indicate that this pattern, consistently cropping up, reflects an incorrect approach to chakra analysis. Hopefully these notes will serve to clarify matters for practitioners who are intent upon increasing their quality of service to those who come to them for help.

CHAPTER SEVEN

INTERPRETATION OF RAY AND CHAKRA CHARTS

Study with care the nature of the rays which presumably constitute the man's nature and provide the forces and energies which make him what he is. I have worded this with care.

Esoteric Psychology Vol. II – Alice Bailey

I would echo, and call your attention to the words – '. . . presumably constitute the man's nature . . .' particularly the word *presumably*. The determination of a patient's rays by radionic or radiesthetic means is a subjective one and thus liable to error. On the other hand it may be a more accurate way of determining them than by directly observing an individual. First of all, direct physical observation to pick out ray characteristics involves time and contact, and even then there may be difficulty in ascribing the ray traits observed or brought out by questioning, to the various bodies. Dowsing used by an informed practitioner obviously has its advantages. It employs the supersensory faculties and provided the practitioner is capable of penetrating the rays as he should be able to penetrate the chakras then a reasonably accurate reading can be arrived at.

In *Radionics: Science or Magic?* I stressed the need to point out to patients that the rays ascribed to them were to be taken only as a guide, as a working hypothesis upon which to base further self-observation, because in the final analysis it is the individual who has to work out his own makeup in terms of energy. So all reports involving ray material are based on the understanding that what is being said is *presumably* right.

I will try to make this a little clearer. We are so conditioned to thinking that black is black and white is white, that we often lack the flexibility of mind to comprehend that at the higher levels of consciousness this may not be so. With rays for example we may find that a person has a preponderance of 2nd ray in their makeup, so much so that we may wonder at their ability to retain good psychological balance. This balance may come from the fact that in their previous incarnation they had a very strong 7th ray trend in their makeup, and in this incarnation it bleeds through and gives them the power to organise and balance which they would not have otherwise had. You may well ask, bleeds through from where? From a past incarnation? Where then are the body or bodies that carried the 7th ray influence? Still around, or are their atoms and particles dispersed back into the pool of substance? I don't know! Perhaps the answer lies in the records held in the permanent atoms, perhaps all time is simultaneous and all incarnations are NOW active. Who knows?

What matters is that if we can present a coherent and fairly accurate picture of the patient to themselves in terms of energy we will be fulfilling our task.

As Alice Bailey says:

> The Science of the Centres is yet in its infancy, as is the Science of the Rays and the Science of Astrology. But much is being learned and developed along these three lines and when the present barriers are down and true scientific investigation is instituted along these lines, a new era will begin for the human being. These three sciences will constitute the three major departments of the Science of Psychology in the New Age . . .

Radionics has pioneered a systematic approach to analysing the states of the chakras and subtle bodies which is something no other healing art can claim to have done. To this we can now add the rays, and when this is done and when practitioners fully understand how to analyse these energy aspects of man, and to make correct interpretations of their findings, then, and only then will radionics achieve its full potential, which after all is nothing more or less than a reflection of the quality the practitioners themselves express from within.

Interpretation is the whole key to this full analysis technique. As I have said before, virtually anybody can dowse out information, but interpretation can only be made in the light of knowledge backed by experience. I am going to repeat a passage from Esoteric Psychology Vol. I at this point in order to set the stage for interpretation and to provide a reminder of just what is involved.

> A ray confers, through its energy, peculiar physical conditions, and determines the quality of the astral–emotional nature; it colours the mind body; it controls the distribution of energy, for the rays are of differing rates of vibration, and govern a particular centre in the body (differing with each ray) through which that distribution is made. Each ray works through one centre primarily, and through the remaining six in a specific order. The ray predisposes a man to certain strengths and weaknesses, and constitutes his principle of limitation, as well as endowing him with capacity. It governs the method of his relations to other human types, and is responsible for his reactions in form to other forms. It gives him his colouring and quality, his general tone on the three planes of the personality, and it moulds his physical appearance. Certain attitudes of

mind are easy for one ray type, and difficult for another, and hence the changing personality shifts from ray to ray, from life to life, until all the qualities are developed and expressed. Certain souls, by their ray destiny, are found in certain fields of activity, and a particular field of endeavour remains relatively the same for many life expressions . . . When a man is two-thirds of the way along the evolutionary path, his soul ray type begins to dominate the personality ray type, and will therefore govern the trend of his expression on earth.

This passage illustrates the importance of ray analysis if you are going to really understand the patient, and through that understanding, help them. It points out the relationship of the rays to the chakras, and that there comes a time when the soul ray begins to dominate the personality ray. Patients who require ray analysis as a guide to help them understand themselves are usually in the midst of the conflict between their personal and transpersonal rays. It is important to be able to intuit where they stand in their development because your interpretation will have to be worded accordingly. This is not always an easy thing to do, but it is an ability that unfolds with practice.

The first thing to note in respect to the patient's rays is the dominance of 1st or 2nd ray traits – does the ray makeup consist of the bulk of bodies being on 1.3.5 or 7th ray, or 2.4.6. Always note the soul and personality rays in particular, and through which aspect of the lower self (mental, astral and etheric bodies) they are working because this is an important factor. A person who has a 2nd ray soul working directly through a ⟨th ray physical will have the capacity to bring the Light of the soul down through to the physical plane in a very useful way because the 7th ray is ever capable of linking the higher to the lower and bringing it through into expression. On the other hand if the physical was 3rd ray this capacity would be somewhat restricted due to the general rule that 2.4.6 work well together and 1.3.5.7 work well with each other – there are exceptions to this as I have already pointed out . . . rays 1 and 2 work very well together on the higher levels of consciousness as previously mentioned, but that combination may not work with such ease and fluidity on the lower astral and etheric levels.

1st ray qualities working together will tend to enhance each other – for example if a person has a 1st ray personality focussed in their 5th ray mind then you can expect an intensifying of both 1st and 5th ray qualities, and it is often the glamours and vices that get heightened and need the softening influence of the 2nd ray. Having said that, a 6th ray personality working through a 6th ray astral body (which is essentially a 2nd ray quality set up) can lead to extreme emotional rigidity and stubbornness, even fanatical attitudes if the vices and glamours come to the fore. If the virtues bloom then obviously the individual is going to be a caring, loyal person – it is a general rule that 2nd ray qualities 'soften' while 1st ray qualities 'harden' attitudes and beliefs.

Each ray has differing effects on the unevolved person and the more highly evolved type. You can as a rule take it that those patients with a life-crisis situation, especially those who are consciously seeking their inner path, will make suitable candidates for this type of analysis. I have never given this matter any special thought, but obviously it does require some discrimination. In my practice I seem to attract a great many patients who are seeking the insight that ray–chakra analysis can give them, and those that don't require it are in a minority.

Before outlining a ray-chakra chart interpretation from my practise I will quote again from Esoteric Psychology II to give a hypothetical ray outline and analysis from the text.

This man has a 2nd ray Monad.

> 1st ray Soul
> 5th ray mental body.
> 6th ray astral body. 2nd ray personality.
> 2nd ray physical body.

Let us see what sort of information this reveals to an initiate.

The second ray quality of his physical body relates him both to the personality and finally the monad. It is, therefore, for him a great problem, a great opportunity, and a great "linking" energy. It makes the life of the personality exceedingly dominant and attractive, and at the same time facilitates the future contact (while in a physical body) with the monad. His problem of soul consciousness will not, however, be so easily solved.

You will note that the monad (2nd ray), the astral body (6th ray) and the physical body (2nd ray) are all along the same line of activity, or of divine energy, creating a most interesting psychological problem. The soul (1st ray) and the mental body (5th ray) are along another line entirely, and this combination presents great opportunity and much difficulty.

In the lower expression of the man whose psychological chart we are considering, the psychologist will find a person who is extremely sensitive, inclusive and self-willed. Because of the fact that the second ray personality and the physical body are related by similarity of ray, there will also be a clearly pronounced tendency to lay the emphasis upon *material* inclusiveness and tangible acquisition, and there will, therefore, be found (in this person) an exceedingly selfish and self-centred man. He will not be particularly intelligent, as only his fifth ray mental body relates him definitely and directly to the mind aspect of Deity, whilst his first ray egoic (soul) force enables him to use all means to plan for himself, and to use the will aspect to acquire and to attract the material good he desires or thinks he needs. His predominant second ray equipment, however, will eventually bring the higher values into play.

In the higher expression of the same man and when the evolutionary cycle has done its work, we will have a sensitive, intuitive, inclusive disciple whose wisdom has flowered forth, and whose vehicles are outstandingly the channel for divine love.

The text goes straight on to point out that:

Many such charts could be drawn up and studied, and many such hypothetical cases could present the basis for occult investigation, for diagram, and for the study of the Law of Correspondences. Students would find it of interest to study themselves in this way, and, in the light of the information given in this *Treatise on the Seven Rays,* they could formulate their own charts, study what they think may be their own rays and the consequent ray effects on their own lives, and thus draw up most interesting charts of their own nature, qualities and characteristics.

Out of the many ray-chakra charts I have done for health care professionals I have chosen one for inclusion in this book. These people are psychotherapists and therefore make ideal subjects for this type of reading, as they are in a better position than most to supply confirmatory feedback in respect to the accuracy of findings and interpretation. One wrote back to say – 'Thank you for your letter. It astonishes me to find descriptions of myself in which I can recognise myself so well!' Another decided to visit me at my office after he had received my written report; I noted as he put the report on my desk between us, that he had ticked off one comment after another. We spent close to an hour going into what the chart reflected, discussing certain points and bringing out things that the written report did not touch upon.

I would add here that written reports are no substitute for a verbal report. Working together on a one to one basis brings out material that would never have surfaced otherwise, and a far deeper insight can be achieved by the practitioner and patient in this context. Normally I will take over an hour to discuss the content of a full radionic analysis, and it is here that a whole new aspect of radionics is waiting to be opened up. The day will come when counselling on the basis of a radionic analysis will be a part of the work – I know that it happens today in a limited way, but the use of ray analysis opens up a field of tremendous potential for radionics, and hopefully in the not too distant future when practitioners have an understanding of the rays and the chakras, this type of work will flourish. In the present crisis of growth that humanity finds itself in, the individual reflects that process on a personal level, and there is a great need at this time for practitioners who can help patients understand the processes going on within them in terms of energy and the way they handle or mishandle it.

The following is a written report on the organ systems, chakras and rays of one of my patients. He is in his late 40's, suffers from asthma which for the most part is not too much of a problem and can be contained quite easily. He is a college teacher lecturing in psychology. I am not going into the organ system imbalances in any detail except to say that the main imbalances showed in the skeletal system (he has some back problems), the sympathetic nervous system, the kidneys and respiratory system. He showed a fairly heavy reading on toxins from chicken pox and aluminium, the latter was no doubt affecting his kidneys. Temperamentally he appeared calm to me and quietly spoken, a certain advantage when working in group situations which he enjoyed doing. So let us look at what his ray and chakra analysis revealed.

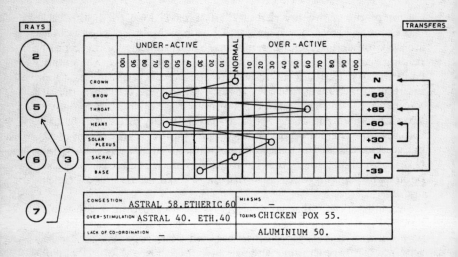

I would like to preface my remarks by stating that it is my firm belief that people who enter the healing/teaching professions along the 2nd ray energy do so, not to teach and heal others but to teach and heal themselves. A real and fundamental inner recognition of this fact, always results in the freeing of the individual from a great deal of the illusion and glamour that surrounds and permeates them. It involves a shift to a higher focus of consciousness, and no amount of intellectual recognition of the real motives for the real reason which they teach and heal will create this shift. It is what Brugh Joy refers to as the 180 degree shift. We shall see that the chakra imbalances and the ray makeup combine to guide the patient into their calling – those in the field of psychotherapeutics will without exception in my experience, show marked imbalances.

The chart shows an abnormally high number of chakra imbalances, but we can expect this in patients who are in the psychological field. My report reads as follows.

Your chakra picture appears to indicate a number of conflicting energy patterns. In fact your chakra readings are quite unusual. Only two of the seven major chakras appear to be functioning within the normal range, the rest are in a state of fundamental imbalance. First let us look at the brow chakra which is the centre of the integrated personality, and governs the pituitary gland, the eyes, ears, nose, sinuses, teeth and brain stem area. As you can see it is underactive, which indicates that the physical organs governed by this chakra are not really getting enough energy, which may to some extent interfere with their full functional integrity. In psychological terms it indicates that you tend to keep the lid on your personality energies, and do not really express them to the full. In short you are introverted rather than outgoing.

Next your throat chakra which externalises as the thyroid and parathyroid glands and governs the vocal and bronchial apparatus, lungs and alimentary tract, is in an over-active state – too much energy is flowing through this centre, and under stressful conditions this will directly affect your lungs and bronchi. Your present loss of voice is directly attributable to this combination of stress and too much energy in the area. At another level this chakra expresses the higher creative energies and the intellect, its overactivity suggests that you in fact employ a great deal of creative intelligence in your work, but I suspect that the underactive brow chakra tends to short circuit some of the expression this should bring into the world around you. The underactive brow combined with the overactive throat indicate to me that you are compensating for imagined personality shortcomings by driving the high amount of intellectual and creative energy you have through the throat chakra – in this way you make up for what you see as personality deficiency.

The throat chakra reflects your desire to be seen and acknowledged, even if your personality is somewhat hesitant about being in the limelight. Your overactive solar plexus chakra which is the seat of the emotional-desire life interacts with the throat chakra so that desire (at the solar plexus level) to succeed drives upward to the throat chakra and brings about the expression of much creative energy. You actualise your creative power through your solar plexus and throat (which upsets your sympathetic nervous system) instead of through your throat and brow chakras. The overload of energy of an emotional type from the solar plexus into the throat relates very directly to your asthmatic trouble.

It is unusual to find an imbalance in the heart chakra, but your heart chakra is underactive, which is interesting in view of the fact that you do a great deal of work in a group context. Such work is of course going to help balance the function of that chakra which is to do with group-consciousness as opposed to self-consciousness in the solar plexus. You can see which dominates, and the indicated path along which you need to progress to open the heart chakra in a proper manner. Its underactive state may reduce your resistance to colds and infectious processes. A full flow of the energy from the heart and throughout the aura is the proper way to keep bacteria and viral invasion at bay. That flow of course, would be reflected in a thymus that did its job properly, as it would if your heart chakra were balanced.

Finally your base chakra which externalises as the adrenal glands and directly governs the spine and kidneys, is underactive. The poor reading on your kidneys is something of an indication of the weakness in the action of this chakra, as are the problems with your spine. Curiously enough it is also a part of your introverted approach to life. Where there is a preponderance of underactive chakras, it is almost always an indication of marked sensitivity, which was too hard to handle in the circumstances surrounding childhood. Too much stress, domineering parents, or too much and too many demands on the individual, can cause them to put up protective barriers by 'shutting down' the chakras and minimising the impact of stressful energies. You have compensated for this by driving your energies through the throat chakra to excel intellectually and academically. The base chakra expresses the physical will-to-be. Its underactive state suggests that there is some reluctance in you to deal with physical plane life, the life of the mind and intellect are far more enchanting, but this will have to be watched because it is a tendency which, if it gets out of hand will deplete your energy at the physical level and loosen your hold on physical reality in an abnormal way.

Your 2nd ray transpersonal self places you on the path of the teacher/healer. While this ray confers the intelligence which you handle with such facility through your 5th ray mind and 3rd ray personality, it can bring with it fears, anxieties, and a poor self-image as reflected in your underactive brow chakra. This ray will not allow you to feel really satisfied with your work, or what you accomplish, no matter how good or effective you are. Work that you do produce will tend to be instructive. It might make you rather cold towards others (underactive heart) or just indifferent at times.

Your 5th ray mind means punctuality is important to you and you are likely to demand it of others. This ray confers common sense which you clearly have in abundance. It gives you independence, a keen intellect, and you will as a rule feel the need to make accuracy count in your work. In some this ray can create an attitude where feelings are rather secondary, combined with the underactive heart it is a point to keep in mind.

Your emotional body is on the 6th ray which will give you an intuitive nature, a strong sense of loyalty and single-mindedness. It also confers feelings that are too intense. which will play havoc through your solar plexus chakra which is wide open and in fact governed by 6th ray energy. This ray can impose a certain rigidity, this in your case reflects into your lung fields and the asthmatic condition. Your 2nd ray transpersonal self is working directly through your 6th ray astral body which means you have the opportunity and the capacity to bring through the energy of love which will touch upon your heart chakra and bring balance to it. Look at your ray chart however and note how the two streams of 2nd ray energy are boxed in by the streams of will energies in your 5th ray mind, 3rd ray personality and 7th ray physical. The latter fortunately will enable you to bring the higher energies down through the physical because it is the nature of the 7th ray to relate the energies of the inner hidden worlds to the physical plane.

The 7th ray governing your physical body should help you to rebalance the base chakra. It confers self-reliance and will make you extremely careful in the details of the work you do. This ray certainly facilitates your teaching and enables you to do so in an ordered manner which students find easy to follow.

Your personality is on the 3rd ray. You will have to watch that this does not lead to too much attention to detail as it interacts with the 7th ray. This is the ray of active intelligence and intellect which is, as we have seen, a dominant theme in your chart and in your life. This, particularly in view of the underactive heart chakra indicates a need to develop the love aspect of your nature, lest hardness, coldness and isolation creep in. This ray gives you an interest in abstract subjects and a capacity to concentrate on philosophic concepts. Your personality is working through your mind or mental body. This coming together of the 3rd and 5th rays will give you a rather strong tendency to be critical of others and even of yourself. Rays 3, 5, 6 and 7 can bring with them a rigidifying influence, and you suffer from rigidity of the rib cage to some extent and especially tightness and tension in the right scapular area. The right side of the body is equated by some schools of thought to the masculine nature, the energy of will. Perhaps that muscular tightness is a symbol of your resistance to the feminine side of your nature and a reflection of the need for the inflow of the softening 2nd ray love energy, with its inclusiveness and openness.

This then is what a ray–chakra analysis report looks like, and it will give you an idea how the material is handled. I subsequently met this patient and we spent another full hour on more details, and in the course of that discussion he confirmed the accuracy of my report. It was my intention to include several such reports, all of which were made for psychotherapists, and all of whom confirmed the accuracy of my outlined findings. However I do not think it will really profit you if I do this – better that you take the data in my books and begin to apply the principles of ray–chakra analysis to your own practises.

I am going to close this chapter with a ray chart for you to peruse. It is worth taking it and figuring out the various combinations of characteristics that would emerge when the soul and personality rays worked through different bodies.

A ray makeup drawn from Discipleship in the New Age, Vol. II by Alice Bailey. This ray analysis was made by the Tibetan Master D.K. for one of his disciples who took part in a group experiment, so it is completely accurate. For those interested there are many such charts to be found scattered in the text. I append below some of the comments made to this person via Alice Bailey.

RAYS

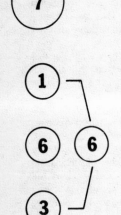

6th ray astral body creates undue attention to details of process, but the 1st ray mind can offset this.

3rd ray physcial inclines to too much physical plane activity, rapid movements and rapid speech.

Tensions constant, too intense, too serious.

Capacity to contact 7th ray soul energies, "banks up" energies in the chakras and galvanises the endocrine glands into activity. This is because there is not adequate use of soul energies.

Energy goes to throat chakra and solar plexus chakra and causes too much vivacious talk.

CHAPTER EIGHT

THE RAYS AND DISEASE

Disease is only a form of transient imperfection.

Esoteric Healing – Alice Bailey

Disease is a complex and very occult process. Its roots lie well beyond the comprehension of man at this time, and we can only theorise as to the root causes which lie aeons behind us before the dawn of time itself. Orthodox medicine sees disease in terms of organ systems and cellular structures, bacteria and viral infections – this physical model of disease is going to rapidly lose validity over the next two decades or so, and predictably will be replaced by one couched in terms of energy. Esotericists have been talking about disease in terms of *too much* or *too little energy* for many years, but the advent of the new physics will bring about the much needed change of direction so needed in the healing arts. Man and his bodies, and the diseases that disrupt and destroy the form, will before too long be seen by science in terms of energy.

Disease is the surface reflection of many things and may be due, from an esoteric point of view to the basic centralisation of life energy, be it in the mental or astral body, the personality or the soul, the head chakras, the solar plexus or the sacral chakra. It may be due to the state of the chakras, congestion or overstimulation of the nadis, earth conditions (geopathic stress), inner tension, inheritance of miasms and genetic imbalances, friction between the soul and personality rays, mental or emotional fanaticism, misuse of sexual energies, inhibited soul energies, a lack of etheric co-ordination and integration, frustration of ideals, a shift of energy from one chakra to another through the internal energy structures. The list is interminable. In radionics we seek the basic causes of disease in a patient, in my opinion whatever the *cause* we pin down in the course of an analysis happens to be, it is not THE cause, but simply a relative one.

By having some understanding of the relationship between the chakras and the rays and between the rays and disease, we can deepen and broaden our understanding of the disease processes in man. Earlier in the book I listed the relationship between the chakras and the ray as follows:

1st ray	Crown chakra
2nd ray	Heart chakra
3rd ray	Throat chakra
4th ray	Brow chakra
5th ray	Sacral chakra
6th ray	Solar plexus chakra
7th ray	Base chakra

Has it occurred to you that this list may be misleading if we don't ask the question, what aspect of the chakras do these rays govern? Is it the mental? I would not think so because we see listed here the chakras above the diaphragm and they do not exist as such at the mental level. What we see listed above are the rays that govern the etheric aspect of the chakras. But what of the astral aspect, which is of vital importance to us because most disease, it appears, originates at the astral or emotional level. So it is necessary to know the rays as they govern the astral matter of the chakras.

1st ray	Crown chakra
2nd ray	Heart chakra
3rd ray	Sacral chakra
4th ray	Base chakra
5th ray	Throat chakra
6th ray	Solar plexus chakra
7th ray	Brow chakra

Here you can see the difference in ray-chakra relationships, and it is important to know this when making an interpretation. Now what of the relationship between the rays and diseases.

1st RAY: CROWN CHAKRA. This ray carries the power to crystalise and make brittle and hard and is related to the atrophying of the physical body, the ageing process which brings about death. It is the ray of the destroyer and related to the disease known as cancer. It is related to self-pity and the sense of the dramatic I at the centre of the stage. Its good aspect lies in sacrifice and the dedication of the I to higher things. Brain tumours are associated with this ray and nerve inflammation. It can also affect the eyes, especially the right one.

2nd RAY: HEART CHAKRA. This ray has great power to build, vitalise and bring coherence to forms. It can easily overstimulate, piling up too many atoms and causing an excessive form of vitality which can adversely affect the bloodstream. The etheric body can become too potent for the physical form and this will result in tumours, growths, cysts, fibroids, supernumerary parts, heart trouble and curiously enough problems concerning the stomach. There is a close relationship in energy terms between the spleen chakra, the heart chakra and the solar plexus – the energies pouring through these centres concerning the life-force will produce tumours, especially if desire and ambition are thwarted or supressed by an underactive solar plexus chakra. Two negative asepcts of 2nd ray energy are self-love carried to extremes, and focus upon and in the personality. At the positive level soul-love and group-love, as opposed to personality-love. People with an underactive heart chakra usually at some level or another have an intense self-preoccupation and lack of group consciousness. On the other hand if the heart chakra is overactive, group consciousness is present and there may be a process of transference of energies into that centre from the solar plexus. In my experience it is rare to find the heart chakra in anything but a normal state, that is functioning within normal limits.

3rd RAY: SACRAL CHAKRA. The 3rd ray is the energy of substance, it is associated with the manipulation of people, situations and energies in an astral manner for material or sexual satisfaction. It will produce intestinal and gastric disorders, stomach trouble, low vitality, certain brain disorders, the so called social dieases, syphilis, gonorrhoea and the present wave of AIDS amongst homosexuals relate to this ray energy. Its negative aspect is over-sexuality and hyperactivity, a so called disease now rampant in children, especially in the United States, the home of AIDS. It may be coincidental but New York city is governed by the 3rd ray and that is where AIDS apparently originated which would make sense in terms of energy. Further to this the personality ray of America is the 6th ray of idealism which relates to the solar plexus chakra and desire, and the soul ray is the 2nd of love-wisdom, an energy that is definitely related to cancerous-like conditions such as AIDS. This disease which is baffling specialists everywhere might just make an interesting study in terms of energy, perhaps before the book finishes I will take a look at it.

4th RAY: BASE CHAKRA. The 4th ray is the ray which diffuses energy, in human terms when energy is diffused it leads to a lack of resistance making it possible for all forms of disease to manifest. Debility can come from this ray, quick and bad reactions to diseases indigenous to the planet – in other words miasms, which may be activated by an intensifying of the flow of this energy through the organism. Falls and emotional shocks also precipitate miasms from the subtle to the physical level, but it is more important to understand the energy dynamics of the process. Great susceptibility to infectious diseases and contagion come from this energy, the 4th ray is behind all epidemics, and influenza is one of its main expressions. Insanity in its various forms is related to this ray. Its negative aspect is dogmatism and selfishness, its higher expression mysticism.

5th RAY: THROAT CHAKRA. This energy demonstrates itself mainly on the mental plane so it becomes the energy associated with many psychological problems and mental trouble. As Bailey points out CLEAVAGE is the outstanding characteristic of this energy, and that cleavage may demonstrate on a personal level between the mental, astral and etheric bodies or between the individual and his group rendering him anti-social. Imbecility is a disease of cleavage are so are many psychological problems. Insanities, brain lesions, certain cancers and metabolic imbalances are 5th ray expressions. Migraine headaches arise as a result of cleavage or lack of relationship between the pituitary and pineal gland energy fields – in other words personality (brow chakra) and soul or spirit (crown chakra are not properly related). Many migraine types have an overactive brow chakra, too much energy through that centre will cause irritation to the pituitary, it swells within the sella turcica and a migraine headache occurs. Some years ago I devised a Rae card to deal with this imbalance which I entitled P-P FIELD HARMONISER, it seems to be effective in some cases and should be used in conjunction with other balancing techniques. One of the negative aspects of the 5th ray is lower psychism, on the higher level its good aspects are creativity, sensitivity and inspiration. Do not forget all of this material is in respect to the astral plane and astral substance, which will reflect into the etheric and finally physical levels.

6th RAY: SOLAR PLEXUS CHAKRA. This energy is related directly to many of the illnesses in the sexual sphere. As Bailey points out, weakness, desire, bewilderment, perversions and the *one pointed* development of sexual focus. Cruelty, lust, sadistic pleasures and sexual diseases arise from the 6th ray energy when its use is perverted. It is also very directly related to gastric trouble, liver disease and diseases of the nervous system. An overactive solar plexus chakra will cause the sympathetic nervous system to become highly sensitized and this in turn will upset the conductivity of the skin – the aura then becomes disorganised and 'open' to invasion from infection and a whole vast array of negative and pathological energies. Emotionalism is the bad aspect of this ray energy, whereas aspiration and right orientation are its positive qualities. Rigid 6th ray attitudes can lead to arthritic and similar joint problems.

7th RAY: BROW CHAKRA. This energy which is now swinging powerfully into manifestation brings together *Life* and *Matter* on the physical plane. It is definitely associated with infections and contagious diseases and promiscuity – it provides the milieu for the growth of bacteria and virus at the lower levels of consciousness and form. Heart diseases and some tumours are related to the 7th ray, as are spinal problems. The bad aspects of this ray are self-interest, pure selfishness and black magic, the good aspect lies in white magic and the manipulation of forces and energies for the healing of man and the planet.

In *Esoteric Healing* we find the following statements:

1. The syphilitic diseases are due to the misuse of third ray energy, that of the creative, intelligent energy of substance itself.

2. Tuberculosis is the result of misuse of the energy of the 2nd ray.

3. Cancer is a mysterious and subtle reaction to the energy of the first ray, the will-to-live, which is one of the aspects of this ray. It works out therefore, in an overactivity and growth of the body cells whose will-to-live becomes destructive to the organism in which they are found.

Syphilis relates to the sacral chakra, the etheric body and the 3rd ray energy.
Tuberculosis relates to the throat chakra, the mental body and the 2nd ray energy.
Cancer relates to the solar plexus chakra, the astral body and the 1st ray energy.

I know that at first sight the concepts I am outlining in this book may seem complex, like some algebraic or mathematical formula. But if you learn the language of the rays and familiarise yourself with their qualities, the time will come when your understanding has transcended the mere learning of the words associated with these energies. Radionics practiced without a good background and understanding of the rays and chakras, is just a pale reflection of the healing art; its potential must be extended into these areas if it is not to crystalise under the impact of the 6th ray energies influencing its practitioners. An extract from *Esoteric Healing* will serve to underline the importance of such knowledge.

These are abstruse and difficult concepts, but they should be pondered upon, and deep reflection will lead to understanding. All disease and ill health are the result of the activity or inactivity of one or other of the seven types of energy as they play upon the human body. All physical ills emerge out of the impact of these imperfect energies as they make their impact upon, enter into and pass through the centres in the body. All depends upon the condition of the seven centres in the human body; through these the impersonal energies play, carrying life, disease or death, stimulating the imperfections in the body or bringing healing to the body. All depends, as far as the human being is concerned, upon the condition of the physical body, the age of the soul and the karmic possibilities.

It is said that there are three primary diseases out of which all others emerge. They are interestingly enough all on the rays of aspect, the 1st (cancer) the 2nd (tuberculosis) and 3rd rays (syphilis). All perceptive practitioners pay attention to the miasms, and I think it is worthwhile at this point considering them in general terms. What is a miasm? When you come right down to it, a miasm is a difficult thing to define in words, and the reason for this I suspect, is due to its very subtle and abstract nature – words don't really define it in realistic terms. Miasms have been defined as energy-patterns of disease, the predisposing patterns of disease, the seeds of disease – whichever way we phrase it the essence of what they are is lost. We shall, for the time being, have to be content perhaps, with the definition of 'energy patterns of disease' but they are much more than that: In esoteric terms they constitute the imperfection of the planetary substance (mental, astral and etheric) from which we draw the material to build our vehicles or sheaths. We attract, according to the programming of substance by the permanent atoms, those materials which may contain the seeds of the three main diseases. The strength of this tainted energy-substance will depend on many factors, suffice to say we choose them, so we are responsible for them and their expression in terms of poor health. If you have a combination of these taints, the tubercular, the syphilitic and the cancerous within the substance of your mental, astral and etheric bodies, it may lay dormant if you live a balanced life. On the other hand the taints or miasms may be activated as previously mentioned by physical and emotional shock, by an influx of a particular ray force, possibly from the soul; or by the ageing process. The result is of course disease, and possibly death which in the final analysis is a transformative process.

What has always interested me is where do these tainted energy patterns reside? I have heard of practitioners who in their radionic analysis work find for example syphilitic miasms on the buddhic plane and higher – let me say here and now this is absolute rubbish, and makes no sense at all if you have any knowledge of these higher levels of consciousness. Some speak of these miasms flowing down from those exalted heights, down through the soul and personality and out into the etheric body of the earth. Into the etheric body of the earth??? for someone else to pick up when they incarnate? I would hope not. Common sense tells us that the miasmic patterns are of a lower order of energy, so it is logical that they will be found imbedded in the attenuated substance of the lower etheric body levels, and the lower levels of the astral and possibly mental bodies. They are comprised basically of 1st, 2nd and 3rd ray energy and those ray energies relate to each of these bodies. Treatment of the miasms must surely be aimed at transformation and transmutation of the tainted substance so that the destructive pattern is unravelled and uplifted and not returned to the earth for someone else to pick up. Esoterically man is upon this planet to transform and transmute the tainted 'soil' of earth at all levels of the three worlds. Channelling miasms back into the earth hardly seems to conform with his spiritual purpose.

The interchange of energy into matter and matter into energy at the etheric and dense physical level holds a clue for us in the handling of the miasms. The atomic elements have a direct role to play in the process of transformation of energy to matter and matter to energy, so in their use lies one of the keys. To this we may add plant and gem remedies according to their rays, and not least of all colour. It is not my purpose to deal with this in detail but simply to point it out.

If we find a miasm in a patient our first instinct is to treat with a view to clearing it out of the system. But is this always the right thing to do? I suspect not, and for a number of reasons. One of these is, that activating the miasm may activate all manner of energy flows that have been damned up on the lower mental, astral and etheric levels. By their very nature and location these energies are likely to give rise to pathological reverberations that might just give the patient a worse set of symptoms to deal with. They may be violently upset both from a physical and a psychological point of view, especially if they are sensitive or getting along in years.

In many instances it is permissible to clear miasms and in the coming chapters we shall consider approaches to this which relate to the ray energies of flower remedies and gems, but I do not envision laying down any hard and fast rules so dear to the hearts of some practitioners.

Hopefully this chapter will underline the fact that the nature of disease is a matter of energy, if we can come to a real understanding of this fact we will have penetrated into the world of causes rather deeply, and this should serve to increase our effectiveness as practitioners.

I would like to return at this point to the subject of the so called social or sexual diseases. Since the liberating energies that made themselves felt in the 1960's we have seen them taken up by many people and channelled through the sacral and solar plexus chakras to create the permissive society. The ensuing over-stimulation has led to an increase in syphilis, the appearance of vaginal herpes, now at epidemic levels in America, and last but far from least, the horrifying disease that primarily affects male homosexuals known as AIDS (Acquired

Immune Deficiency Syndrome). This disease attacks its victims by depressing the functions of the immune system to the point where it barely works at all, the result is the individual has no resistance to infections of a bacterial, viral or fungal nature. A rare form of cancer then appears known as Kaposi's sarcoma which produces frightening skin lesions, inevitably pneumonia makes drastic inroads into the victim's rapidly decimated health, weight loss occurs and eventually the victim dies. There is no known cure for this disease and it is highly transmissible from person to person or through blood transfusions.

It appeared to begin simultaneously in New York, Los Angeles and San Francisco, since then it has spread rapidly throughout the country and overseas to other nations. It has been linked to drug taking which would transmit the disease through the communal use of dirty needles used to shoot up drugs. But it seems that the disease can strike non drug uses, heterosexuals and people who don't need blood transfusions, as do haemophiliacs. Three million Americans each year require blood transfusions, and should one of them be transfused with AIDS infected blood, the effect is terminal.

If you think about it this disease is a terrifying spectre, it can take from six months to three years to incubate, and many people might have the disease long before it makes its appearance. The effect upon individuals within the homosexual community has been mixed – it ranges from sheer terror to a suicidal don't-care attitude, in many instances it drives homosexuals into a state of celibacy, which when you consider that the average AIDS victim had sixty different sexual partners over a twelve month period, means that a lot of energy is going to be blocked, and that in itself will bring on psychological and physical disease. Before looking at the ray and energy aspects of this disease it is worth considering some statistics in respect to the sexual revolution. It is believed that as many as 20 million Americans suffer from genital herpes, which is incurable by scientific orthodox means, but non-fatal. There are an estimated 1 million new cases of gonorrhea and 100,000 new cases of syphilis reported each year. As you can see the permissive society has managed to produce some startling statistics, and no doubt a great deal of suffering and distress.

A number of research laboratories in America are trying to unravel the baffling mystery of AIDS, spending in the region of tens of millions of dollars to track down the causative factor which from a mechanistic orthodox point of view, has to be a virus or bacteria of some kind. What I would like to do in the context of this book, is to look at the sexual diseases in general and AIDS in particular, from the point of view of ray energies and chakras. Exercises of this kind can enhance our capacity to grasp the objective, surface phenomena and penetrate to the energies that lie behind them.

The medical model of reality demands that a physical cause be sought for any disease, and so naturally all research into this disease will flow along such lines, but let us look at it from a vibrational energy point of view. AIDS apparently appeared simultaneously in New York, Los Angeles and San Francisco, from an energy point of view it is most likely to have originated in New York which is the throat chakra of the American continent, and on the 3rd ray which is the ray associated with syphilitic and social diseases of this kind. I would suspect that from there it flowed naturally to Los Angeles which is the heart chakra, governed by the inclusive magnetic pull of the 2nd ray. I do not know if San Francisco is classified as a chakra, but if my memory serves me rightly Chicago is the solar plexus of America and New Orleans the sacral chakra, which are governed by the 6th and 5th rays respectively. AIDS may well have gone to Los Angeles via Chicago because the solar plexus energy is attracted to the heart. Irrespective of this, I find it interesting that New York being on the 3rd ray is the most likely point of origin for AIDS.

If we look at the chakras of man that play prominent roles in this disease we have two primary pairs. The sacral and throat chakras, representing the sexual or lower creative energies and the higher creative energies of the throat, and the solar plexus chakra and the heart chakra. The former is the centre of the instinctive desire-life, while the heart is its higher counterpart which interestingly enough governs the thymus gland, a vital aspect of the immune system. Linked very directly to the heart and solar plexus by energy channels is the spleen chakra which pours the life force into the organism to directly vitalise the physical form via the blood stream.

The average citizen will quite probably be amazed at the number of sexual partners a homosexual may have, many it seems had up to 1,100 different partners on a lifetime average. Can you envision the amount of sexual and desire energy that this must involve, and the effect that this profligacy must have upon the chakras, not only below the diaphragm but also on those above? It is impossible to escape the consequences of such misuse of energy. The sacral and solar plexus chakras are going to become highly overactivated, and this enormous amount of energy is going to be driven upwards into the heart and throat chakras, disturbing lung and alimentary tract function for a start, not to mention that of the thyroid. The heart, overburdened with polluted energy will in turn affect the physical organ, the thymus, the circulatory system and not least the blood.

In terms of the ray energies involved with these chakras we have the following to consider.

The sacral chakra. Etheric aspect, 5th ray of the lower mind.

Astral aspect, 3rd ray of active intelligence.

Sexual diseases are part and parcel of the misuse of 3rd ray energy, and relate to sexual satisfaction, the manipulation of others and low vitality.

The Solar Plexus chakra. Etheric aspect, 6th ray of devotion.

Astral aspect, 6th ray.

This means that the solar plexus chakra has a very potent 6th ray quality, and energy which is directly related to sexual diseases, weakness, desire, bewilderment which grows out of misdirected desire and perversions. So you see already just how the look at AIDS is coming together in terms of ray energies.

The chakras above the diaphragm that are involved are the:

Throat chakra. Etheric aspect, 3rd ray of active intelligence.

Astral aspect, 5th ray of the lower mind.

So the same rays govern the sacral and throat chakras, the 3rd and the 5th, but please note that they govern different aspects which sets up a strong polarity and pull. The 3rd ray is as we have already seen associated directly with social diseases and the 5th ray imbalance will bring about metabolic disorders, mental problems and some forms of cancer.

Heart chakra. Etheric aspect, 2nd ray of love-wisdom.

Astral aspect, 2nd ray.

Again a double power of the 2nd ray. Now consider what diseases are related to this energy. In the earlier part of this chapter I indicated the power of this ray to vitalise and bring coherence to forms – it can easily overstimulate and pile up too many atoms in a given area and this bunching up of atoms inevitably produces forms which we know as tumours. It also generates a peculiar form of vitality which has a very insidious affect on the bloodstream, and which also creates tumours. Add to this the life force pouring in through the spleen chakra and you have a recipe for disaster.

One need hardly say anything further, already in terms of energy you have an aetiology for this disease that has only one antidote, and that is normal sexual relationships. For the victims of course, that path or way out is shut until life is terminated by death and reopened by rebirth in a future experience.

In *Esoteric Psychology Vol. I,* Alice Bailey writes:

Man has to learn and deeply grasp the fact that the main purpose of sex is not the satisfaction of the appetites, but the providing of physical bodies through which life may express itself. He has to understand the nature of the symbolism underlying the sexual relation, and by its means grasp the scope of spiritual realities.

Elsewhere in the same volume we find:

These perversions are ever found when a civilisation is crumbling and the old order is changing into a new.

As to the esoteric causes of homosexuality, they lie in a combination of a very active sacral chakra combined with a not so active throat chakra. The upward movement of sacral energies unable to flow into the throat chakra find a place in the heart centre where they are temporarily retained. This can result in stimulating the sex urge, religious eroticism, and unwholesome attitudes ranging from fanatical celibacy to sexual perversions of all kinds of homosexuality. Bailey points out that homosexuality is a left over, a taint rather like a miasm, from the sexual excesses of a previous civilisation.

Of the mechanics in terms of energy she states:

In those days, so urgent was the sexual appetite, the normal processes of human intercourse did not satisfy the insatiable desire of the *advanced man* of the period. Soul force, flowing in through the processes of individualisation, served to stimulate the lower centres. Hence, forbidden methods were practised. Those who thus practised them are today, in great number, in incarnation, and the ancient habits are too strong for them. They are now far enough advanced upon the evolutionary path so that the cure lies ready at this time – if they choose to employ it. They can, with relative ease, transfer the sex impulse to the throat centre, and thus becoming creative in the higher sense, employing the energy sensed and circulating in right and constructive ways.

If one reads the reports on AIDS victims and the homosexual communities' reaction – the cry is for more research to find a cure for the disease – what they are looking for is a chemical cure so that they can continue the old lifestyle without any of the risks. This disease is so virulent and so fundamental a perversion of the use of energy that it is doubtful if a cure or vaccine of this kind will emerge.

In Romans I the initiate St Paul writes of these problems, and if you read what he writes in terms of energy you will see that he knew what it was all about. To the Biblical text I will add my own comments, in brackets and italics.

22. Professing themselves to be wise, they became fools,
23. And changed the glory of the incorruptible God into an image made like corruptible man, and to birds, and fourfooted beasts, and creeping things.
24. Wherefore God also gave them up to uncleanness through the lusts of

their own hearts *(heart chakra)*, to dishonour their own bodies between themselves.

25. Who changed the truth of God *(the higher expression of the ray energies)* into a lie *(the lower expression)* and worshipped and served the creature *(low-self: personality)* more than the Creator, *(High-Self, Monad)* who is blessed for ever. Amen.

26. For this cause God *(Monad)* gave them up to vile affections: for even their women did change the natural use into that which is against nature:

27. And likewise also the men, leaving the natural use of the women, burned in their lust *(2nd and 6th ray energy)* one toward another; men with men working that which is unseemly, and receiving in themselves that recompense of their error which was meet.

28. And even as they did not like to retain God *(Monadic and soul energies)* in their knowledge, God gave them over to a reprobate mind, to do those things which are not convenient:

Thus the Biblical text goes on. A fundamentalist would see the social diseases, particularly AIDS as a punishment from God, such simplistic interpretations do not in any event apply. When man breaks the Law of his own Being down through the ages, he sows the seeds of his own destruction in himself. Sooner or later they are going to germinate and give rise to painful reminders that we ourselves are responsible for our lot, and that we have the power within to change it from a corrupt imbalance of forces and energies to a glowing and radiant reflection of Truth.

It had been my intention to write only a few lines about the social diseases but my thoughts on the subject have traced their own path. These diseases reflect in a stark and graphic manner just what happens when energies associated with the lower chakras are manipulated and misused. I think too it illustrates how useful a subtle energy model can be in looking at man and disease, and for that matter health, in a different light.

CHAPTER NINE

GEM REMEDIES AND THE RAYS

The note of the mineral kingdom is the basic note of substance itself.
Treatise on Cosmic Fire – Alice A. Bailey

Minerals have held a fascination for man down the ages, and he has used precious and semi-precious stones for decorative purposes, to heal sickness and to ward off detrimental influences. The mineral kingdom carries a whole variety of energies which can be used for therapeutic purposes, naturally these are ray energies so we shall look at them from that angle. In this manner I will deal with seven gemstones only, but I hope that from this will come some new insights as to how they can be employed in the light of our knowledge of the rays, subtle bodies, chakras and disease.

The mineral kingdom is directly influenced by the 7th ray of Organisation and the 1st ray of Power. The secret of this kingdom is said to lie in the process of Transmutation, which can be defined as the passage across from one state of being to another through the agency of fire, both literally and in terms of energy. For this reason, I believe that the Gem Elixirs will prove of great use in the treatment of miasms, particularly when related to flower remedies on the same or similar rays. Bailey points out that the healers on the 3rd ray can best employ the use of remedies made of herbs or minerals belonging to the same ray as the patients under treatment. This approach would certainly add an important and vitally new dimension to the whole practice of homoeopathy, and to radionics.

In *Spiritual Body and Celestial Earth,* author Henry Corbin writes at some length on the Sufi metaphors for the subtle bodies, and the inner alchemical processes which transmute dense silica and potash into the opacity of glass through which the inner hidden things can now be seen. The process of refinement proceeds through glass to crystal, and when a magical white Elixir is added to the crystal it takes on the property of now being able to set things on fire. The process then moves by mysterious means to produce diamond from the crystal. Corbin writes:

And diamond, freed from crystal, freed from glass, freed from stone, corresponds to the believers bodies in this absolute Paradise.

How well that passage reflects the 1st and 7th ray qualities, the organising and transmuting power. Bailey points out that the various mineral substances fall into seven main groups which correspond to the rays, and that powerful hidden changes take place in the mineral kingdom when, and only when the 7th ray is in manifestation. Well it is coming into manifestation now, although it still has to contend with the influences of the outgoing 6th ray which we see so clearly illustrated for us in the state of the world today, and not least in organised radionics, but 6th ray rigidity will have to give way to the transformative and transmutive power of the 7th, and in this process we shall see gemstones emerge into prominence in the healing world.

The mineral kingdom in its own way shows a very advanced state of spiritual development which is reflected in its radiatory power. Radium is evidence of this, and it took the psychic sensitivity of two 7th ray disciples, the Curies, to intuit this and make the discovery known to science at a terrible cost in physical terms to themselves. The 7th ray is one of ritual and organised form, thus the energies in the mineral kingdom are very directly related to geometrical patterns. We can assume with little fear of contradiction that Malcolm Rae was a 7th ray disciple who brought his systematic mind to bear on the problems and mysteries of radionics, certainly the geometric patterns he devised were a reflection of his 7th ray qualities. Malcolm, if anything, was the most systematic man I have worked with in radionics, and there can be no doubt that the cards he developed and the simulators he invented to focus their organising patterns will be with us for a long time to come, and they will continue to play an increasing role in homoeopathy and radionics.

It may be of interest here to list the divisions of the mineral kingdom and their correspondence to consciousness.

1. Base metals ....Physical plane. Dense consciousness.
2. Standard metals ....Astral plane. Self-consciousness.
3. Semi-precious stones ....Mental plane. Radiant consciousness.
4. Precious jewels ....Soul consciousness and achievement.

Now let us look at the seven gems that correlate with the seven rays. I will take them in order and outline each one and its therapeutic uses individually. These correlations are drawn from the teachings of Theosophy in general and from the writings of Geoffrey Hodson in particular.

FIRST RAY: DIAMOND

The diamond is said to be the enemy of the Devil because it resisted his power by day and night. It is said to endow the wearer with superior strength, courage and fortitude. Some thought it to be a stone of great power and could drive away nocturnal spectres. Curiously enough it is a stone often associated with thunder and lightning, and an anonymous Italian manuscript asserts that diamonds were sometimes consumed or melted by thunder and lightning. One can't help wondering if that manuscript was actually dealing with some esoteric facts couched in metaphor when you consider that two of the names given to the 1st ray are:

The Lightning which annihilates
The Power that touches and withdraws
or for that matter:
The Fiery Element, producing shattering

Remedies made from diamond are said to be an antidote for poisons, they were used to treat bladder problems especially where calculi were involved. It was used as a protection from plague or pestilence, and in cases of insomnia.

SECOND RAY: SAPPHIRE

The sapphire was thought to be a powerful defence from harm, and capable of attracting divine favour. Like the diamond it was thought to be an antidote for poison and bring good luck. The star sapphire has been called a "Stone of Destiny" because the three bars that cross it are said to represent Faith, Hope, and Destiny. Therapeutically it is thought to have been useful in removing impurities from the eye, and for treating diseases of the eyes. There are records which show that it was thought to be efficacious in the treatment of plague boils.

THIRD RAY: EMERALD

This stone was said to improve supernatural powers and to enhance and even confer prophetic powers. It was used to strengthen memory, or enhance the eloquence of speech, sharpen the wits and quicken the powers of intellect. Magicians used emeralds to strengthen their spells and to give them the power of fore-knowledge. Like many stones it was used as an antidote for poisons and for wounds that were poisonous. Many used it as a protection against demoniacal possession. Paracelsus recommended it for treatments of the eyes. In India it was used as a laxative, and elsewhere to treat epilepsy, fever, haemhorrhages and leprosy. If placed upon the stomach it helped gastric and liver complaints. The ancients also used it in cases of haemoptysis.

FOURTH RAY: JASPER

Jasper has been credited with the capacity to bring rain, and drive away evil spirits. Some claimed that it literally withdrew snake poison from a bite, into itself. Jasper is the gem of Libra and a symbol of St Peter.

FIFTH RAY: TOPAZ

Based on the affinity of planets to stones, Paracelsus claimed that topaz was related to Jupiter. It was the symbol of St Matthew and strongly recommended by St Hildergard to cure dimness of vision. Like the sapphire, topaz was also used in the treatment of plague sores and boils.

SIXTH RAY: RUBY

The wearing of a ruby is said to assure the individual concerned of a life lived in peace and concord, preserving them from all danger and peril. This stone would also guard the house, orchards and vineyards from damage by high winds. It was considered by Naharari, a 13th century physician of Cashmere, to be useful in the treatment of flatulency and biliousness. Some physicians on the basis of *similia similibus curantur* used the ruby to treat haemorrhages and all inflammatory states and to remove anger and discord.

SEVENTH RAY: AMETHYST

Traditionally amethyst was used to cure drunkenness. Some claimed that it controlled evil thoughts and protected from contagion. In an old manuscript it states that if a bear is engraved on an amethyst it will keep the wearer in a sober state and puts demons to flight.

I have listed the rays and the gemstones attributed to them, and then added just a few details drawn from various sources. These details were not meant to be of any particular use from a therapeutic point of view. While a lot of the claims made for the curative properties of stones sound far fetched, and some of them probably were, the fact remains that there was and still is validity in the concept that gem stones do have therapeutic and protective properties which can be used. It seems that ideally such stones should be in direct contact with the skin to have the maximum effect.

At the beginning of this chapter I mentioned that the mineral kingdom is governed by the 7th and 1st rays. To us the radiations from radium are very apparent, but those from gemstones are not at all so obvious. With the increasing influence of the incoming 7th ray there will be a corresponding increase in the radiatory effect of gemstones, and I am certain that with the right research through radionics a lot of interesting work in this area will be forthcoming.

The rays listed for each of the gemstones are the primary ray assocated with them, obviously there must be other ray influences in them just as there are people and plants, but in the lack of any real knowledge on this subject we shall have to be content with knowing the main ray influence that each carries and expresses. Certainly for therapeutic purposes this will suffice.

There are any number of books now appearing on the market about gems and gem therapy, and the worldwide interest in the healing power of crystals is our response to the increasing tide of 7th ray influence that is flowing through man and this planetary system. As this power intensifies so will the power inherent in the crystal increase along with the potency of radionics as a diagnostic and therapeutic procedure.

CHAPTER TEN

FLOWER REMEDIES AND THE RAYS

The vegetable kingdom has a peculiar place in the economy of the system as the transmitter of the vital pranic fluid; the vegetable kingdom is definitely a bridge between the conscious and the unconscious.

A Treatise on Cosmic Fire – Alice Bailey

While the mineral kingdom is influenced by the 7th and 1st rays along the line of Will, the vegetable kingdom comes under the influence of the 2nd and 4th rays along the line of Love. These bring respectively, increased sensibility and harmonisation. To the governing 2nd and 4th rays is added the 6th ray of devotion. The line of 2.4.6 is ever the line of the healer and plants have been used for thousands of years, not only to sustain the life of humanity but to heal its ills.

Bailey lists the *secret* of the plant kingdom as follows:

Transformation. Those hidden alchemical processes which enable the vegetable growths in this kingdom to draw their sustenance from the sun and soil, and to "transform" it into form and colour.

The *purpose* of the plant kingdom is:

Magnetism. That inner source of beauty, loveliness and attractive power which lures the higher forms of life, leading the animal forms to consume it for food, and the thinking entities to draw from it inspiration, comfort and satisfaction of a mental kind.

You will perhaps have noted that three rays govern the plant kingdom while the mineral has only two. The reason for this is the advanced point of evolution this kingdom has reached along its own path of spiritual development. Man is also governed by two rays, those of the soul and personality until he approaches the final leg of the evolutionary journey, at this point the monadic ray begins to make itself felt, and then three rays govern.

In the plant kingdom the 6th ray governs all aspects of the trees that populate the planet. The 2nd ray expresses itself through the beneficent influences of flowers and cereal plants, and the 4th ray through the grasses and smaller life-forms. Dr Edward Bach must have had a strong line of 2nd, 4th and 6th ray. He was a highly sensitive person which was a reflection of his 2nd ray, this gave him the capacity to sense the vibratory healing qualities of the flowers, so much so that he actually experienced the moods and fears that each plant would help to alleviate. He was very one-pointed and determined to carry out his work with plants despite the fact that the Medical Council threatened to strike him off their list. Bach's 6th ray idealism and devotion comes through clearly, as do his intuitive powers. No one was going to tell him what to do once he had found this important aspect of his life's work, not even the Medical Council. The fact that he destroyed a great deal of material, and left little about himself indicates the glamour of the 2nd ray, self effacement to an excessive degree. I feel too that he must have had a 4th ray in his makeup, giving him a great love of colour and beauty. It is interesting too that he found the vibratory stress of life in London very distressing, and this forced him into the countryside and into the most important phase of his work. People with a lot of 2nd ray qualities in their makeup have great difficulty in coping with crowded and stressful places because they absorb so much of the surrounding impressions that they can be overwhelmed by them at times.

Before dealing with the ray influences in the Bach Flower Remedies, I want to digress for a moment to write about the California Flower Essences and the work of Richard Katz and Patricia Kaminski in California, who with a group of colleagues and helpers have thoroughly researched and put together several Flower Essence Stock Kits. Stock Kits 1 and 2 contain 24 essences each and range through a whole variety of flowers. The Flower Essence Society produce one of the most beautiful and professional journals I have seen in a long time, and it reflects the thoroughness and sheer professionalism of their approach to healing through flowers. The Journal has now given way to a Newsletter which is a pity, but nevertheless it is highly informative and indicates the vitality of their work. I would strongly recommend anyone to subscribe and to begin using the Flower Essences.

Each Flower Essence has listed with it certain qualities and patterns of imbalance that it is good for. I would like to list several to give you an idea how this looks – I personally find it most useful following a full radionic analysis, to radionically determine those Flower Essences which reflect the patient's life lessons and patterns of imbalance. Let me show you one or two examples.

PLANT	LIFE LESSONS AND INNER QUALITIES	PATTERNS OF IMBALANCE
California Poppy	Psychic opening, spiritual balance, integration of past life abilities and knowledge, spiritual sight.	Blockages of creativity and intuition, externalisation of spiritual goals.
Penstemon	Inner strength through adverse circumstances.	Self-doubt, feeling over-whelmed by challenges, adversity.
Self–Heal	Self-healing power of self-acceptance and self-trust, being nourished by life energy.	Self-doubt, confusion.
Yarrow	Protection from harm by the strength of one's inner light.	Vulnerable to psychic or emotional "attack", to harmful environmental influences or energies.

Some of the essences in the first two stock kits are Lotus, Zinnia, California Wild Rose, Shasta Daisy, Quaking Grass and Manzanita. All twenty four essences can be purchased along with coloured photographs of each flower with an affirmation relating to the healing properties the essence contains. I especially like this addition because it is a fact that positive health affirmations serve to enhance the benefits of any remedy we may take.

The following are examples of some of the affirmations used.

CALIFORNIA POPPY
I am clear and balanced in my spiritual and psychic unfoldment.
I am awakening abilities and understandings from deep within my being.
I see clearly with my spiritual sight.

PENSTEMON
I persevere patiently through difficult situations.
I have the inner strength to overcome frustrations and obstacles.

SELF-HEAL

I accept the self-healing power within me.
I am confident and clear.
I receive nourishment from the life energy around and within me.

YARROW

I am emotionally strong, unaffected by the emotional pull of others.

Affirmations such as these are a potent adjunct which will enhance the effects of the essences being taken. In the Summer 1980 issue of The Flower Essence Quarterly, editor Richard Katz writes:

> Flower essences and affirmations are both potent ways of transformation, and their combination can be potent indeed – a co-operation of the creative power of the conscious mind with the subtle catalytic action on the vibrational level of the essences. While it may be true that flower essences can affect us independently of our beliefs, their effects can be greatly enhanced by cultivating beliefs which affirm the qualities and changes we seek.

Even a cursory glance through the Flower Essence Quarterly back issues, clearly reflects the vital new energy and the expansion that this California based group have brought to this area of treatment. While the group have initiated careful research and exploration into the use of native flower essences they have not forgotten the work of Edward Bach from which they drew inspiration. In fact it is clear that what they have done, without disturbing the original concepts of Bach, is to expand upon his work in a dynamic and most positive manner. If you have ever harboured any doubts as to the efficiacy of flower derived remedies, the articles, so beautifully presented in the Quarterly would erase them in short order. I would urge any practitioner to join the Flower Essence Society, learn about the California Flower Essences from their writings. The information available will give you new insights into the use of flower essences and remedies, and add a whole new dimension to your diagnostic and interpretative abilities.

While we in England have plodded along with true British reserve in our use of flower remedies, the Californians have added a dynamic sparkle and a quality of enthusiasm which we tend to lack on this often overcast island. Like the work done in radionics with the chakras, subtle bodies and rays, there must be a vital and enthusiastic belief in the whole approach, based on sound knowledge, and applied with certainty and confidence. A lack lustre attitude of, oh well, try this and see if it works! is just not good enough. The energy of our belief and enthusiasm must be employed to back up the subtle healing vibrations of the flower essences and remedies, thus creating a true co-operative relationship between us and the deva essences we are working with – there really is no other way to go about this work.

I see the work of Richard Katz and Patricia Kaminski as a sound and essential extension of Edward Bach's ideas, and this whole new dimension breaks through the limitations set upon Bach's works in some quarters. Certain authorities believe that Dr Bach did all there was to do in the field of flower remedies – that the work begins and stops where he began and stopped, this is a typically 6th ray crystallised attitude, which encourages entrenchment into the past and a blinkered view of the world of flower remedies. The Californians by their very nature have injected a stream of positive 2nd and 4th ray energy, carefully balanced by the 7th ray of order. Get in touch with their work and you will see what I mean.

They have also devised affirmations for the Bach remedies, and these as you will see in a moment, provide a new dimension to their use. One of course does not have to use just these affirmations, it is quite in order to formulate your own, but be sure that they are statements of a positive nature. Don't say – this is getting rid of my weakness, because this, in a very real sense is acknowledging weakness. Say instead – this is strengthening me in every way.

SCLERANTHUS
I am decisive in thought and action.
I am balanced and stable.
I act from inner certainty.

OLIVE
I feel revitalised in mind and body.
I make conscious use of all my energy.
I tap into an unlimited energy source within me.
I know my limits in sharing with others.

WALNUT
I am free of limiting influences.
I follow inner guidance despite other's influences.
I am protected from any negative influence.
I break all links which hinder my growth.

These last two affirmations are surely ideal for the radionic practitioner to employ on a daily basis. Because of the constant inter-relationship between the patient and practitioner at the higher and lower levels of the personality, and the pathological energies involved this form of protective affirmation can be very useful.

FULL LIST OF CALIFORNIA
FLOWER ESSENCES AND THEIR RAYS

STOCK KIT No. 1

FLOWER ESSENCE	RAYS	FLOWER ESSENCE	RAYS
Blackberry	2-4	Pink Yarrow	1-3-5
Borage	3-6	Red Clover	2-4-7
California Poppy	2-4-6	Sagebrush	1-3-5
Chamomile	2-3-5	Scarlet Monkeyflower	3-6
Dill	3-5-6	Scotch Broom	2-4-6
Fuschia	4-6	Self-Heal	2-4-7
Iris	4-6	Shasta Daisy	1-3
Madia	5-7	Star Tulip	2-4-6
Manzanita	2-4-6	Sticky Monkeyflower	2-4-6
Morning Glory	2-4-7	Sunflower	2-4
Nasturtium	2-4-5	Sweet Pea	4-7
Penstemon	2-4-6	Yarrow	2-6

STOCK KIT No. 2

Basil	1-3-4	Larkspur	1-7
Black-eyed Susan	3-4-7	Lavender	3-7
Bleeding Heart	4-6	Lotus	1-2-3
Buttercup	2-7	Marigold	2-7
Calif. Wild Rose	2-4-6	Pomegranate	1-3-6
Cayenne	1-2-4	Quaking Grass	2-4-6
Corn	2-5	Rabbitbrush	2-4
Dandelion	2-6	Saguaro	3-5-7
Garlic	1-5-7	Saint John's Wort	2-5-6
Golden Ear Drops	2-5	Trumpet Vine	2-6
Goldenrod	2-3-6	Yerba Santa	6-7
Indian Paintbrush	3-5	Zinnia	2-3-6

From these lists and the ray lists of the Bach Flower remedies, it is possible to develop a ray-chakra-flower essence approach to prescribing, which should prove both interesting and effective.

FLOWER ESSENCE QUALITIES: STOCK KIT No. 1
Stock Kit No. 1 is comprised of 24 flower essence prepared in North

America by Richad Katz. During the last five years its use has spread throughout the world, and it has rapidly acquired an impressive reputation for effectiveness.

BLACKBERRY *Rubus ursinus* (white-pink): conscious manifestation using the creative power of thought; for overcoming inertia or feeling stuck.

BORAGE *Borago officinalis* (blue): cheerful courage, confidence in facing danger and challenge; for overcoming discouragement or grief.

CALIFORNIA POPPY *Eschscholzia californica* (golden orange): balanced inner development, intuitive and creative abilities; for overcoming spiritual "glamour" and over-fascination.

CHAMOMILE *Anthemis cotula* (white/yellow centre): inner calm and objectivity, release of emotional tension; for nervousness, insomnia, emotional upset; good for children.

DILL *Anethem graveolens* (yellow): assimilation of experience; for feeling overwhelmed and overstimulated by the pace of life.

FUCHSIA *Fuchsia hybrida* (red-purple/pink): awareness and understanding of blocked emotions; for repressed emotions often expressed as tension, illness, or false emotionality.

IRIS *Iris douglasiana* (blue-violet): artistic and creative inspiration; for overcoming feelings of frustration and creative limitation.

MADIA *Madia elegans* (yellow/red spots): concentration, focus, attention to detail, follow-through; for the tendency to be easily distracted or side-tracked.

MANZANITA *Arctostaphylos viscida* (white-pink): appreciation of the physical body and world; for ambivalence or negative judgement of the physical.

MORNING GLORY *Ipomoea purpurea* (blue): vitality, alertness, help in breaking old habit patterns; for restlessness, jitteriness, erratic energy.

NASTURTIUM *Tropaeolum majus* (orange-red): earthy expressiveness, vitality; for over-intellectuality or devitalization.

PENSTEMON *Penstemon davidsonii* (violet-blue): inner strength through adversity; clarity and relationships; for self-doubt when faced by challenges.

PINK YARROW *Achillea millefolium* var. *rubra* (pink-purple): emotional strength and balance; for overcoming emotional oversensitivity and reactiveness.

RED CLOVER *Trifolium pratense* (pink-red): centredness and balance in emotionally charged group situations.

SAGEBRUSH *Artemisia tridentata* (yellow); being true to one's essential self: letting go of what is inessential or excess, releasing false self-images or expectations about self.

SCARLET MONKEYFLOWER *Mimulus cardinalis* (red): courage to work with powerful emotion, with the "shadow" side of self; emotional balance.

SCOTCH BROOM *Cytisus scoparius* (yellow); motivation, perseverance, acceptance of difficulties as opportunities; for overcoming pessimism and despair.

SELF-HEAL *Prunella vulgaris* (violet): self-acceptance, trust in inner health-creating forces.

SHASTA DAISY *Chrysanthemum maximum* (white/yellow centre): synthesis and integration of ideas into a unified understanding; for those with a tendency to scattered seeking.

STAR TULIP *Calochortus tolmiei* (white-violet): inner sensitivity and receptivity, inner listening.

STICKY MONKEYFLOWER *Mimulus aurantiacus* (orange): awareness of sexual issues, integration of sexual and love feelings; overcoming fears of intimacy.

SUNFLOWER *Helianthus annuus* (yellow): developing individuality; overcoming egotism or unbalanced self-effacement; harmonising inner relationship with father principle.

SWEET PEA *Lathyrus latifolus* (red-purple): social responsiveness and rootedness; overcoming social alienation or conflict, and fears of social commitment.

YARROW *Achillea millefolium* (white): strengthening of one's inner light in relating to negativity or disharmony; for over-sensitivity or feeling vulnerable.

FLOWER ESSENCE QUALITIES: STOCK KIT No. 2

Stock Kit No. 2 is a revised version of the FES Research Kit, used by hundreds of FES members the past three years.

BASIL *Ocimum bacilicum* (white): integration of sexual love and spirituality; helps penetrate to the core of emotional issues between people.

BLACK-EYED SUSAN *Rudbeckia hirta* (yellow, black centre): penetrating insight, emotional transformation.

BLEEDING HEART *Dicentra formosa* (pink): releasing emotional attachments; brings peace, harmony, balance to the heart.

BUTTERCUP *Ranunculus occidentalis* (yellow): knowing the value of one's gifts; sharing one's light with others; for shyness, withdrawal.

CALIFORNIA WILD ROSE *Rosa californica* (pink): vitality, rejuvenation; love of life.

CAYENNE *Capsicum annuum* (white): catalysing quick change, for overcoming ingrained habits.

CORN *Zea mays* (yellow-white): spiritual roots, balanced

relationship between Heaven and Earth; emotional detachment and clarity; helpful in dealing with crowded environments.

DANDELION *Taraxacum officinale* (yellow): cutting through emotional blockages; releasing tension.

GARLIC *Allium sativum* (white): releasing fears; overcoming insecurities, nervousness.

GOLDEN EAR DROPS *Dicentra chrysantha* (yellow): gaining perspective on unhappy childhood memories.

GOLDENROD *Solidago* sp. (yellow): owning one's power with others; being true to one's self in relating to others; letting go of barriers to interpersonal contact.

INDIAN PAINTBRUSH *Castilleja miniata* (red): awakening the vitality of the creative impulse; gaining emotional maturity by working through frustrations.

LARKSPUR *Delphinium depauperatum* (blue-violet): generosity, altruism, true leadership qualities.

LAVENDER *Lavendula officinalis* (lavender-violet): inner peace through self-appreciation and spiritual self-knowledge; harmony through spiritual thoughts.

LOTUS *Nelumbo nucifera* (pink): spiritual tonic, enhances essences and practices; overall balance.

MARIGOLD *Tagetes erecta* (yellow): inner listening; hearing others; hearing the child within us.

POMEGRANATE *Punica granatum* (red): freeing feminine creative energy (in men or women); finding how to express one's creativity; helps transform emotions relating to lack of childhood nurturance.

QUAKING GRASS *Briza maxima* (green): group harmony and co-operation; blending of individual egos.

RABBITBRUSH *Chrysothamnus nauseosus* (yellow): alertness, sharp awareness, overview of all detail.

SAGUARO *Cereus gigantus* (white, yellow centre): clarity in relation to parental/authority images; appreciating the wisdom of true spiritual elders and tradition.

SAINT JOHN'S WORT *Hypercium perforatum* (yellow): releasing conscious and subconscious fears; trust in spiritual protection and guidance; helps deal with fearful dreams.

TRUMPET VINE *Campsis tagliabuana* (red-orange): vitality in self-expression; self-assertion.

YERBA SANTA *Eriodictyon californicum* (violet): spiritual insight into emotions; relaxation of emotional constriction, especially around the heart.

ZINNIA *Zinnia elegans* (red): laughter, lightness and release of tension; child-like playful attitude toward life; accepting the inner child.

As well as being given orally these flower essences can be 'broadcast' or projected to the patient at a distance using the Bervroux Compass. The pattern is oriented N–S and the patient's witness placed at the center. Phials of the appropriate remedies are then placed on the point ascribed to their fundamental ray and the length of distant treatment dowsed for.

CALIFORNIA FLOWER ESSENCE KIT I

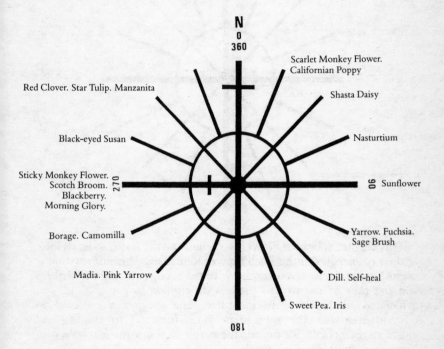

CALIFORNIA FLOWER ESSENCE KIT II

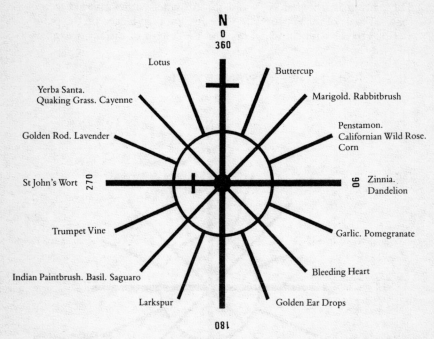

This chapter is headed Flower Remedies and the Rays, so let us look at the ray energies of the Bach Flower Remedies. This information is useful in that it can be correlated with the rays governing the chakras and the rays of the patient to provide a guide to prescribing. The associated tissue salts are identified, and these can be used in combination with the appropriate Bach remedies to amplify and augment their effect. We can add the astrological sign too for those who bring this aspect into their work.

SIGN	TISSUE SALT	BACH REMEDY	RAYS
Aries	Kali Phos	Walnut	1st 6th 7th
		Wild Oat	1st 6th 7th
		Crab Apple	1st 6th 7th
Taurus	Nat Sulp.	Elm	1st 4th 5th
		Rock Water	1st 4th 5th

Gemini	Kali Sulph.	Agrimony	2nd 3rd 4th
		Water Violet	2nd 3rd 4th
Cancer	Calc Sulph.	Pine	3rd 6th 7th
Leo	Silica	Cherry Plum	1st 2nd 5th
		Rock Rose	1st 2nd 5th
		Oak	1st 2nd 5th
		Chicory	1st 2nd 5th
Virgo	Nat Phos.	Larch	2nd 5th 6th
		Holly	2nd 5th 6th
		Cerato	2nd 5th 6th
		Olive	2nd 5th 6th
		Gentian	2nd 5th 6th
Libra	Calc Fluor.	Chestnut Bud	1st 3rd 5th
		White Chestnut	1st 3rd 5th
		Scleranthus	1st 3rd 5th
		Aspen	1st 3rd 5th
		Star of Beth.	1st 3rd 5th
		Impatiens	1st 3rd 5th
Scorpio	Kali Mur.	Centaury	4th 6th
		Wild Rose	4th 6th
		Mimulus	4th 6th
		Vervain	4th 6th
Sagittarius	Mag Phos.	Willow	4th 5th 6th
		Mustard	4th 5th 6th
Capricorn	Calc Phos.	Sweet Chestnut	1st 3rd 5th
		Clematis	1st 3rd 5th
		Gorse	1st 3rd 5th
Aquarius	Nat Mur.	Honeysuckle	4th 5th 7th
		Red Chestnut	4th 5th 7th
Pisces	Ferr Phos.	Beech	1st 2nd 6th
		Vine	1st 2nd 6th
		Heather	1st 2nd 6th
		Hornbeam	1st 2nd 6th

These correlations come from the book *Esoteric Healing – Flower Remedies and Medical Astrology* by Dr Douglas Baker, B.A., M.R.C.S., L.R.C.P., F.Z.S. and is one of many excellent books he has written on esoteric matters. Dr Baker is a leading authority on the writings of Alice

Bailey and a highly accomplished esoteric astrologer. I realise that some of the sign–tissue salt correlations do not agree with those traditionally given but this may well be due to the esoteric viewpoint from which they have been made.

It should be apparent from this material on the California Flower Essences and the Bach Flower Remedies that we have in these ethereal medicines, potent tools of healing, especially if used in the light of our knowledge of chakras, rays and subtle bodies.

CHAPTER ELEVEN

GEOPATHIC STRESS AND EARTH ENERGIES

> To come face to face with the Earth not as a conglomeration of physical facts but in the person of its Angel is an essentially psychic event which can "take place" neither in this world of impersonal abstract concepts nor on the plane of mere sensory data.
>
> *Spiritual Body and Celestial Earth* – Henry Corbin

In his book Corbin goes on to say that the Earth has to be perceived not by the senses but by or rather through a primordial image. Our earth, from an esoteric point of view, is indeed considered to be a living entity, an angel if you like, but an imperfect one, thus its energies have both beneficial and destructive effects.

Over the past decade or so the concept of ley lines and sacred alignments between ancient stone sites and many churches, has become common knowledge thanks to the books of John Michell and others. Radiesthetists and dowsers in general have long been aware that certain areas of countryside give off energy patterns which are inimical to health. Even orthodox medical records and statistics show that there is a correlation between certain geographic and geological areas and the incidence of specific diseases.

Before looking at the more material aspects of this subject, I want to quote at length some passages from *Esoteric Healing* by Alice Bailey.

> I shall, and can, say but little – only enough to indicate one fruitful cause of disease and one of such great age that it is inherent in the life of the planet itself. These diseases have no subjective or subtle origin; they are not the result of emotional conditions or of undesirable mental processes. They are not psychological in nature and therefore cannot be traced to any activity of the centres. They originate from within the planetary life itself and from its life aspect, having a direct emanatory effect upon the individual atoms of which the dense physical body is composed. This is a point of importance to remember. The source of any disease of this nature induced by the planet itself, is due primarily, therefore, to an external impact of certain vibratory emanations coming from the surface of the planet, engendered deep within the planet, and impinging upon the dense physical body. These radiations play upon the units of energy which, in their totality, constitute the atomic substance of the body; they are unconnected in any way with the blood stream or the nervous system. They are consequently impossible to trace or isolate, because man is

today so highly organised and integrated that these external impacts immediately evoke a response from the nervous system; the modern physician is at present unable to distinguish between the diseases arising from within the patient's own interior mechanism – tangible or intangible – and those which are in the nature of extraneous irritants, producing immediate effects upon the sensitive organism of man's body. I am not here referring to infectious or contagious difficulties.

Perhaps one point which I might helpfully emphasise is that it is this obscure planetary effect (obscure to us at this time) upon the physical body which is the major cause of death where the purely animal form nature is concerned, or the forms of life present in the animal and vegetable kingdoms, and to a lesser and slower degree in the mineral kingdom likewise.

This passage holds a number of clues as to the nature of this apparently destructive radiatory energy coming from the earth itself. If it deals out death to the atomic structures of the physical body then it may well be in some way associated with the energies of the 1st ray. Whether this idea will be of any use to us I do not know. What I do know is that dowsers have for years known about negative energies in the earth which can arise it seems from underground streams, geological faults, tunnels, mines and ley lines.

French radiesthetists coined the term for this malefic energy, they called it VERT NEGATIF or NEGATIVE GREEN. This band of radiation is located in the colour spectrum between the colours white and black, and will kill bacteria and mummify meat. The French, Chaumery and Belizal in particular, one of whom incidentally is said to have died due to his researches into radiesthetic energies, wrote of the negative green band as a "noxious wave" – they subdivided this band into *Alpha waves* emanating from subsoil cavities and geological clefts. *Beta waves* from contaminated currents of water, sometimes known as 'black streams' from subterranean water-flows. *Gamma rays, Theta, Nu and Zeta waves* which come from ordinary radioactivity or harmful radiations coming from television sets, or the wiring of the house itself which can affect some people adversely.

Enel, a famous radiesthetist who worked along the lines laid down by Chaumery and Belizal, did a vast amount of research into the Vert Negatif energy and specialised in treating cancer patients with it. He finally contracted the disease himself, and in his opinion there was no doubt that he brought it upon himself by passing the energy through his body when using the spun pendulum technique for treating patients. Incidentally Negative Green is the energy of pyramid fame, so we may wonder about the advisability of sitting in pyramid shapes during meditation. If Negative Green energy mummifies meat and other products, do we really know what it does to the human body in the long term? I doubt it.

Research in France led to the discovery of "cancer houses" which got this designation when it was discovered that literally every apparently healthy family that moved into them and lived there for any length of time, inevitably had members who succumbed to cancer. Radiesthetic checks indicated strong sources of Negative Green radiations under these houses that brought death in their wake. Here perhaps is another indication that these planetary radiations are 1st ray in nature, because the 1st ray is related to cancer and to the process of death or abstraction from form.

While Bailey says in her treatise on the rays and healing that these energies are not detectable, perhaps after all they are, and if progress in the field of energy medicine is anything to go by there are now objective techniques for identifying their effects in patients. In my office I use the Vegatest methods of diagnosis which have grown out of some twenty years of research into electro-acupuncture started by Voll in Germany. The Vegatest method can amongst other things detect pre-malignant states, measure the functional integrity of all the organ systems, determine specific types of psychic stress and interestingly enough – geopathic stress, which is the name given to those radiations that emanate from the interior and surface of the planet. The Vegatest protocol recognises five kinds of radiation which it deals with under the heading of geopathic stress. These are:

> Yin – discharging force fields
> Yang – charging force fields

The former is identified as coming from running underground water, caves, mines, geological faults. Some 80% of all geopathic stress comes from these sources. The Yang charging force field can come from mineral, salt, oil or ore deposits. This accounts for some 20% of all cases. Radioactivity seldom occurs according to Dr H.W. Schimmel, M.D., D.D.S., who originated the technique – certainly it can show up in a radionic analysis as witnessed by the patients I have cited elsewhere in this book. Then there is:

> Global grid stress

This is due to ley line activity and shows up quite clearly if present when using the Vegatest technique. Then comes:

> Radioactive stress

and

Electromagnetic disturbances

These two are self explanatory and arise from nuclear radiation or from electrical sources such as power lines running overhead and the wiring in the house.

Medical research using the Vegatest shows that patients suffering from geopathic stress have gone from doctor to doctor seeking help but to no avail. They are often the perennial patients who no one seems able to help. The reason for this is THAT PATIENTS SUFFERING FROM GEOPATHIC STRESS WILL NOT RESPOND TO ANY TREATMENT UNTIL THE SOURCE OF THAT STRESS HAS BEEN DEFUSED OR THEY MOVE TO LIVE ELSEWHERE.

When I first came into radionics, John Damonte a radionic practitioner and an authority on radiesthesia, put great store into determining the presence or absence of Negative Green energies in his diagnostic work, and incidentally he was another practitioner who fell victim to the energies handled in this field, and died prematurely. One way or another I learned a lot from John, but I notice nowadays you hear little or nothing about Negative Green energies upsetting patients. Perhaps as a result of its undetected presence there are practitioners banging their heads against the wall trying to get people right.

There are a number of techniques used to 'clear' or dampen down these negative energies coming from the earth. One is to detect the line of energy running under the house and to drive in metal rods beyond the confines of the building, rather like acupuncture treatment of the earth. Another method is to wind copper coils and place them in strategic positions. I recently did a radionic analysis in which the patient concerned had a very marked set of organ imbalances as well as subtle body and chakra problems. I detected geopathic stress. Subsequently a request for a diagram of the ground floor plan of the house showed an overground sewer pipe running directly beneath the house, under the bed in the bedroom, and then under the kitchen sink. This source of harmful radiation was damped down with copper coils wound around the pipe at the point before it entered under the house and where it emerged. The patient confirmed that she had never felt really right since moving there eight years previously.

Psychic stress like geopathic stress will nullify any treatment that is not aimed directly at it. By psychic stress I mean all heavy daily stresses that impinge upon the personality at all levels. These have to be dealt with by using the California Flower Essences, the Bach Flower Remedies and a variety of Gem Elixirs designed to balance the subtle bodies and chakras, with special attention to the astral body and the solar plexus chakra.

I suppose we can include the pathological states that arise from metallic toxins in this chapter, but I will only list them briefly to call your attention to them, becuase like geopathic stress, if the source is not removed health will not improve. Some of these sources of toxins are mercury-silver amalgam fillings in teeth, which can upset health to a marked degree as toxins from the mercury and other alloys leach into the body. Included at the end of the book is an article on this that appeared in Radionic Quarterly. This will give you further information. Aluminium toxicity from cooking utensils is a prime source of poor health in people who are sensitive to this metal. I had colitis for five years as a result of aluminium cooking ware being used in my home when I was a child.

Perhaps we have strayed a little from the subject of earth energies, but I hope that what I have written will alert you to their dangerous aspects. Obviously there are magnetic spots on this earth which are the source of fine healing power, but we have to become aware of both the positive and negative aspects of the radiations that radiate from the living body of this planet earth.

Miasms seem to be impregnated into the very substance of the earth, and their detection in radionic work has always been important. During the writing of this book I happened across an article on the miasms written by the late John Damonte, which he gave to me sometime during the early 1970's. Reading through it I decided that it would be a shame for this material to lie unused in my files, because it provides an excellent insight into these disease bearing patterns, which I am sure will be of use to practitioners. The full text of John's article including his original heading, comprises the following chapter, I have simply added the lead-in quotation.

CHAPTER TWELVE

A STUDY OF THE MIASMS FOR RADIONICS

The reduction of the sum of human karma through the experience of this planetary war (1914 – 1945) will enable the souls seeking incarnation to create bodies free from tendencies to morbid developments.

Esoteric Healing – Alice Bailey

Greater success in radionic assessments can be achieved with a foreknowledge of the homoeopathic principles of the miasms.

The dictionary defines miasms as: "A poisoning of the air by germs or harmful particles", but the word will be employed here in its homoeopathic sense. In homoeopathy miasm denotes a transcending and predisposing condition that causes illness.

We should therefore consider contagion, incubation and evolution as a modification of the life force. If we view the miasm as a four dimensional dynamic encompassing the vital force, the mind (psyche), the body (soma) and the species, there was neither spontaneous cure nor natural ending without some stereotyped long term changes in successive generations.

This can be understood further when we regard an illness as an imbalance of the vital force and can perceive when there are disturbances in the physiological and anatomical continuity of a live organism. These disturbances are nothing less than symptoms; groups of symptoms of a determined order and identified with a cause are syndromes. In point of fact pathology describes syndromes only.

Since an unwell person presents a syndrome that has the characteristics of being conditioned by a specific keynote, we could safely say that the makeup of every individual is governed by his own species and his own intrinsic nature.

The ideas of diathesis, constitution and morbid predisposition suggest to us that symptomatology, apart from the syndrome that labels it, depends in some constant way on the individual's makeup or his individual mode of reaction. During an acute illness this individual mode of reaction should overcome any non-lethal crisis. It is convenient to say, therefore, that a symptomatology, even one which corresponds to tissue destruction, represents an effort of the individual's vital force to adapt itself to a new situation by seeking an equilibrium. The illness represents a compound of symptoms having some relation to the disturbing cause and with a disproportion that is in favour of the vital force. Combining these ideas, we could equate the individual's mode of reaction with the individual's vital force.

Thus in our approach to sickness we must consider both the cause of the disturbance and the individual's mode of reaction or vital force, with all their characteristics. The course and the eventual disentanglement of a sickness depends on the achievement of an effective equilibrium between the cause of the disturbance and the individual's mode of reaction. This mode of reaction has two salient features: the general ability to react against the disturbing cause and the individual method of so doing. In addition, the causes of disturbance also present two features for consideration: their power and their duration. When a cause of disturbance is weak or brief and/or when the vital force is capable of effective balancing up, the result will fall within the symptomatic cycle (regardless of its name) that will present a beginning, a period of fluctuation and an evident end. This describes an acute condition known as cyclic illness. When the cause of the disturbance is of an undefined intensity but of long duration and/or when the vital force is weak, we are faced with an acyclic illness, better known as a chronic condition. Hahnemann states that chronic diseases are due to the infection of an existing chronic miasm. He also means that any measure of infection or contagion of a chronic disease should be regarded from a dynamic viewpoint before being regarded from the bacteriological viewpoint.

THE MIASMS

These are three in number: psora, syphilis and psychosis.

Psora is the fundamental miasm, being the oldest contagion of the vital force, the "superior" cause that inhibits or reduces the mode of rection of the dynamism. Syphilis and psychosis have no precedence over one another, but exist in conjunction with psora. There is no syphilis except syphilis-psora. There is no psychosis except psychosis-psora. It is probable that we may observe pure psora in the course of time.

Each miasm is an old contagion. Once the miasm has affected the vital force it has a stationary period with a localised manifestation which, more often than not, gets suppressed. Then the miasm affects deeper spheres and multiple symptoms begin which can give a false appearance of being unconnected with the miasm. From that moment on, the vital force becomes a tributary to the miasm, bearing its seal, whilst retaining its own individuality. Two results arise from this: the heredity factor of the miasm in the period of evolution and the stable symptomatic framework (miasmatic syndrome). We must also bear in mind that the miasm diffuses itself among the species producing a multitude of aspects, observable in different individuals. In order to understand its manifestations, it is necessary to be acquainted with all the symptomatology of the homoeopathic remedies that are anti-miasmatic. The chronic case can only show a small pattern of the whole mosaic.

In order to achieve a stable cure, one must appreciate, know, study and identify the miasms.

Briefly,

1. Miasms constitute the basis of every chronic condition, always being determined by the constitution and temperament of the individual.

2. Miasms spread out among the generations of the species.

3. Miasms, being of an infectious, contagious nature, are dynamic and can only be extinguished dynamically.

4. The most important of the miasms is psora, which lies beneath any illness and lends foundation to it.

5. In treatment, the last miasm to disappear is psora.

6. When the morbid framework is a complex of three miasms, its cure can become impossible when we find, in addition, some other 'miasm' of medical origin (here 'miasm' is used academically) such as vaccinosis, toxins, poisons, viruses, etc.

7. Syphilis and psychosis take root in psoric terrain.

8. Miasmatic contagion is of a dynamic nature, i.e. there would be acarus in a psoric skin, neisseria in a psychotic mucous and treponema in a syphilitic mucous.

   There are sufficient foundations to presume that miasms are contagious.

9. The miasm has its seat in the dynamic, expressed in the body and transcends the psychic sphere.

10. In practice, one should not forget that a miasm is a constitutional state resulting from anti-natural suppressions.

PSORA

Psora is a great disorder of the vital force, the pathological keynote of which is pruritis (the perennial itch as I like to think of it), going from the most superficial areas to the deepest ones of the organism, from the vesicle or blister, to symptoms of anxiety and epilepsy, passing through a multitude of psychopathological malfunctions. It is the most ancient and widespread miasm affecting humanity, the most contagious in its superficial manifestations and the most versatile. In various periods of history, it has suffered a change due to suppression of its primary superficial expressions, which suppression has occasioned deeper expressions affecting organs and vegetative functions. In the past the deepening of this miasm was caused by accidental means more or less logical at the time, such as thermal waters followed by use or abuse of metals and metalloids as the basis of externally applied remedies. We can appreciate that today this deepening of the miasm is even more prevalent due to the use of alcaloids, antihistamines, hormones, antibiotics, X-rays etc., both as therapy and for purposes of diagnosis. Taking into account these new methods, it is logical that new forms appear in men today rendering the task of homoeopathy more difficult in assessing the similimum. Therefore, radionics as well as radiesthesia becomes a necessity to homoeopathy, providing, of course, we keep to a method of approach that is unhindered by external agencies. We should not fall into the trap of chasing 'red herrings', but should remain concerned with the chain of Cause and Effect as we are now aware of the four-dimensional character of the Primary Cause.

As an aside, I would like to say that in my radionic assessment, I always like to interrogate the patient so as to earmark the clinical antecedents, his past symptoms and sicknesses, his psychological make-up and the hereditary factors and vectors, whenever possible. Then I envisage the possibility of neutralising and balancing the toxicity resulting from his present medical condition. The aforementioned factors could come under what has been termed earlier as an 'academic' miasm. For these we have wonderful and proven homoeopathic remedies such as potentised antibiotics, bowel organisms nosodes and specific drainers. I have personally used radionic pointers such as special rates covering the psychic spheres and the psychological spheres, in quickly administered tests. All these factors, when strongly established, can render someone refractory to radionics in the same way that they have rendered people refractory to homoeopathy and allopathy.

At this juncture I should like to add the following advice:

Radiesthesia is detection at a distance. Radionics is action at a distance.

Whilst detection is in some cases physical and in others mental, it is the detector's intellectual equipment that is going to govern his degree of accuracy in detection. The sum total of the unfathomable source of knowledge of the collective unconscious is there, available to all detectors. Nevertheless, the greater the detector's mental 'capital', the better will he be able to create a narrow 'radar beam' to the collective unconscious to get the most correct answer. As this also applies to radionics for action at a distance, any questions that could have arisen are now answered by: 'good dowsing, well timed and well directed'. By the same token, one can find more accurate and universal rates chiefly when the principle evoked is subjective, as for psychic and mental rates.

To conclude these remarks, let me comment on further aspects and symptomatology of miasms. To recognise a dominant psoric we must investigate its first appearance, bearing in mind that is is only a part of the primitive condition and that there are also the aggregate symptoms corresponding to its progress or to the addition of other miasms.

In the dominant psoric, we would discover symptoms in their latent forms, arising from multiple functional changes in the internal organs, and others that confirm the existence of deep cellular modifications, having the effect of producing defective assimilation of the constitutive elements of the cells and being the basis of various degenerations well recognised in anatomopathology (or biology).

The Psoric-Syphilitic: This disequilibrium is a fundamental modification that afflicts the psoric, the keynote of which, in addition to the existing insufficiency, will now have the element of destruction in the dynamic as well as in the corporal spheres over a wide range of types from the psoric–syphilitic to the syphilitic–psoric in accordance with the dominant psychosomatic factor in each particular case.

The Psoric-Psychotic: This is another modification which produces exaggeration in the productive and possessive sense, together with disquiet and anxiety and precipitance, both mental and physical. This combination will also present a wide range from the psoric–psychotic to the psychotic–psoric. Thus, at first sight, a psoric would appear to be underfunctioning generally, emaciated and reticent, or he would be fat with flabby flesh, pale, slow, inhibited by anxiety or fear. Should he display more apprehension and anxiety or restlessness, or be more extrovert, then we have on our hands a psoric with a psychotic modulation. If, on the other hand, he is aggressive, mistrustful and reticent, he would be a psoric with syphilitic modulation.

SYPHILIS

In homoeopathy this miasm is the result of obstruction of the natural function of the skin in producing sufficient antibodies for general organic protection. Medication eventually proves inadequate as a morbid constitutional condition ensues, expressing itself as a strong imbalance of the vital force, with destructive tendencies both in the soma and the psyche.

Clinical evolution could be described as follows: After contagion, the spirochaete swiftly invades the bloodstream and the lymphatic system, the lesion appearing within ten to ninety days at the place of contagion or inoculation. This primary lesion has the appearance of an indurated, indolent protuberance with an indented summit. It is commonly known as a chancre and is accompanied by hypertrophy of the lymphatic ganglions and would be so located as to be unobservable, for example, in the female genital organs.

In the context of Hahnemann's medicine, the chancre presents a second disorder in an individual who already possesses the first disorder (psora). Because it is of a distinct nature, it is susceptible to an evolution of its own and presents secondary and tertiary conditions. (For further details refer to medical works describing the complete clinical aspects).

PSYCHOSIS

The word 'sycosis' is derived from the Greek 'sycon' meaning a wart or excrescence.

Psychosis is a clinical reality and expresses itself in hyperfunctions such as catarrhal and eliminative eruptions of the skin, the mucous membranes, the digestive system, the respiratory and urinary systems. These eruptions may be accompanied by sclerosis, arteriosclerosis and the production in the skin, mucous membranes, and viscera of benign or malignant tumours such as excrescences, condyloma, melanomas, warts, adenoma and neoplasm.

Its origin is gonorrhoea and here again it superimposes itself on psoric terrain and thereby affects the vital force.

Research has been made on this miasm and several conflicting conclusions have been arrived at. Be that as it may, we shall remain with the homoeopathic concept which I consider sufficient in its present form for radionic radiesthetic purposes.

BASIS FOR CLASSIFICATION

In general when classifying any symptoms one should bear in mind that anything that indicates insufficiency or defects relates to psora-, anything that indicates perversion or destruction relates to syphilis-, anything that manifests excess, exuberance or hyperfunction relates to psychosis.

The psoric is reflective and his characteristic slowness gives him time to be so. The syphilitic is destructive. The psychotic is harried, the basic disquiet of the miasm leading him to behave in this way; he is extrovert and ostentatious.

The psoric is anxious but can dissimulate; he appears to be waiting for something that never arrives but which he nevertheless needs. The syphilitic is harassed; this state is deeply rooted and of long duration; he cannot hide his feelings; treatment with drugs or even with homoeopathic similes can make the miasm clear up. The psychotic expresses pure fear and is disquieted by nature; his nervousness causes him to fear the worst.

The psoric is timid, the syphilitic is cruel and the psychotic ambitious; the first because of his slowness and introversion and the dominance of the 'hypo' factor; the second because of his marked tendency to destroy; the third because of the dominance of the 'hyper' factor.

The psoric is slow, sometimes careless and sometimes mutinous and this applies to all his functions. The syphilitic is easily upset, passion offends him and he is capable of the worst type of acts. The psychotic acts nervously and precipitately.

In the face of danger, the psoric inhibits and paralyses; the syphilitic attacks even those stronger than himself, the stress being on destroying or being destroyed; the psychotic hesitates, withdraws and thinks afterwards that he could really have confronted the situation.

The psoric is sad and depressed in accordance with the keynote of the miasm. The syphilitic is a sentimental–passionate type and his disordered feelings can lead him towards destruction, even his own. The psychotic seems distressed and must be so because of his dominant physical and mental unrest.

The psoric is irritable and ill-humoured because of his unsatisfied needs-, the syphilitic is choleric but quick to please; the psychotic is irascible, rude and ill-mannered but quickly retracts or apologises in order to compensate the hyperfunction.

In a delinquent act such as a robbery, the psoric will plan the robbery, the syphilitic will attack the guard and the psychotic will effect the robbery; the first because he is reflective and a thinker and cannot steal (unless he is psoric-psychotic); the second because of his destructive tendencies; the third because of his ambition to possess.

The psoric lover is more mental and contemplative (masturbation is a hallmark of the psoric); the syphilitic can spend his time thinking of sex and fall into the worst perversions (destruction of the species); the psychotic is sensual and given to sexual excesses, and he is cynical and likes to boast about his successes.

The memory of the psoric is poor. He understands well what is said or what he reads but finds it hard to memorise. However the data remains once memorised. The syphilitic does not remember recent happenings but retains remote incidents in their chronological order (this shows the truly deep roots of the miasm which conserves past incidents). The psychotic, because of his precipitate approach, has an active memory and records everything. He has discernment to evaluate what is worthwhile memorising but is impatient to sit down and study.

The psoric is tired of his physical ups and downs which lead to further deficiencies of all types, especially if only the symptoms were handled, whether by homoeopathy or by radionics. The syphilitic is disappointed as his condition tends, by its very nature, to worsen, especially if some ulceration has been suppressed; from disappointment he can go to despair. The psychotic has a very active mind and he tends to exaggerate greatly.

The psoric tends to be mentally confused; he is always wiser after the event; he can argue well in writing. The syphilitic will present mental lapses during aggravation of the miasm. The psychotic is quick in his repartee, dangerous in argument, but lacking in depth. His disquiet obliges him to participate in everything and he takes on more than he can handle.

The psoric can think of death but will never reach the point of suicide. The syphilitic thinks of death, his own and that of others . . . . but he is capable of hiding his feelings and will not speak about it, hence his suicide can be a surprise to all. The psychotic could, by nature, commit suicide. He will advertise his intentions and will manage to have someone around to rescue him in time.

The following traits can also appear in the three miasms:

Aggressiveness: The psoric can be aggressive when no other recourse is left to him. The psychotic can be aggressive and will keep up a pretence of courage in public but will also be prompt to retract or make amends. The syphilitic is aggressive because of rancour and hate.

Jealousy: The psoric underestimates himself whilst he overestimates the loved one. The syphilitic is basically jealous with disregard for self and for the object of his jealousy. He can kill or commit suicide and can kill his loved one or her seducer with premeditation, knowing full well the punishment he will receive. The psychotic is sure of his superiority over any rival and considers undignified any attention by others upon the object of his love.

Alcoholism: It seems obvious that the syphilitic should have the monopoly of this tendency, but any other miasm can have it. The psoric alcoholic drinks for the purpose of filling a need, but will only drink alone or with very trusted friends because of his natural timidity. The syphilitic drinks because of his tendency to self-destruction and is the most difficult alcoholic to cure. The psychotic can drink a lot and may boast about his ability to hold his drink. He may be the kind of host that invites friends and exhibits a roll of notes to pay the bill.

Sleeplessness: The psoric cannot sleep because of abundant ideas; the syphilitic because of tormenting ideas; the psychotic because of mental and physical disquiet.

Dreams: (The following are only examples). The psoric forgets his dreams and tends to dream just on the point of waking up. The syphilitic has dreams of murders, accidents and absurdities. The psychotic has pleasant dreams of banquets, money, changes or location;

these dreams seem true on waking up; he can also have anxious dreams.

Digestive System: The psoric does not assimilate well (hypofunction). The syphilitic has a disorganised digestion. The psychotic is overnourished (hyperfunction).

Other Physical Functions: The secretions of the psoric are serious; those of the syphilitic are bloody; those of the psychotic are purulent (putrid). The menses of a psoric woman would appear to be of small duration and/or retarded; those of the syphilitic would be irregular both in quantity and frequency; those of the psychotic would be abundant and/or painful.

Urinary System: In the psoric the urinary system is liable to present arduous micturition, the aggravation being inflammation due to some obstruction. In the syphilitic the obstruction will present ulceration that could cause dysuria and bloody urine. The psychotic will tend to have an abundant micturition with a tendency to be fetid; the obstruction will be through tumours.

Respiratory System: The psoric will have clear mucous and phlegm. The syphilitic will reveal blood in his expectoration and suffer from nosebleeding. The psychotic will be characterised by his tendency towards colds and sinusitis. The tubercular person is predominantly psoric; he will be psychotic-psoric or syphilitic-psoric according to whether he has proliferative or destructive tendencies. Tuberculosis does not present us, therefore, with sufficient independent conditions to be considered as a miasm. It is a condition like any other bacterial condition and its malignancy depends on the miasmatic background. However, because of the subtleness of radionic assessment, I am rather inclined to include tuberculosis as a miasm (in the academic sense). I am concerned here with remanence and hereditary conditions for diagnostic, prognosis and research purposes.

Skin: The skin of the psoric will exhibit pruritus with non-purulent and bloodless secretions. The syphilitic will have blood in his secretions. The psychotic will have suppurating infections with various types of excrescences. Tumours are basically sycotic but will become malignant only through the combination of the three miasms, making the prognosis dependent on the predominant miasm. A cancer case, basically psoric, will live longer, the symptoms remaining mild; he will think that his condition cannot be remedied. The syphilitic cancer case will die as the result of cellular destruction. The psychotic cancer case will have a massive and swift invasion. Here again, cancer need not be considered as an independent constitutional miasm, and what has been said earlier on about tuberculosis applies.

Modalities: Each miasm has its own characteristics. The psoric can experience aggravation at any time of day or night, whilst the worst moments are around 12 noon. The syphilitic is at his worst at night. The psychotic ameliorates when the sun sets. Cold will aggravate the psoric; heat, the syphilitic; changes of temperature, the psychotic.

Other Peculiarities Relating to Ages: The newly born psoric can have a delicate skin, wide fontanelle, rather a big head and contract rashes and dermatitis. He perspires when eating and has a lazy digestion. He will feel better for perspiring and he likes being covered. The newly-born syphilitic could present malformations. He tends to have umbilical bleeding and he can have a jaundiced appearance. He sleeps in the daytime and he cries and perspires at night. The perspiration does not get better and he prefers to be uncovered because of his preference for the cold. The newly-born psychotic can have eye conditions and he is prone to infections. He perspires easily when covered up and displays a lazy respiratory system. He will show a tendency to want to uncover himself when asleep; in sleeping, too, he manifests disquiet.

Later on the psoric will not assimilate well and will present problems when weaned; the problem is not so much the choice of diet as the innate nature of the child. The syphilitic will have difficulty in suckling, has a good appetite and tends to prefer anything that has already proved unstable; his stools are fetid, perhaps with signs of blood. The psychotic eats well and gains weight; his stools and micturition are abundant and he is vulnerable to changes of temperature.

The pre-school child appears subdued and easily handled when he is psoric; he is destructive when syphilitic; he is restless and uneasy when psychotic.

The psoric schoolchild is slow to memorise and needs to work harder than the others, but he will retain well once he has learnt his subject; he tends to be clumsy and below average in games and sports. The syphilitic schoolchild asserts himself; he has filthy habits and would be cruel to animals or weaker individuals. The psychotic schoolchild will obtain good marks even when working less than others; he is content to make the grade; he is good at games and sports and he generally loves physical activity.

The teenage psoric has difficulty in adapting; he tends to be introverted and puberty is his most difficult period. The teenage syphilitic will create all sorts of juvenile problems and tends to scorn authority to the point of rebellion. The teenage psychotic will have problems in making a specific goal; he will try everything without persistence and he will even abandon schooling to earn money; he is a typical 'builder of castles in Spain'.

The older psoric will have a dry, weathered skin; he is sad in old age and feels misunderstood. He is obstinate and will atempt to impose his conservatism on his progeny whilst awaiting death patiently; his end is marked by organic underfunctioning and hypotension. The older syphilitic is a nonconformist, opposing everything and everyone and making life insufferable for those is his environment. His end is marked by ulcerations of all sorts and he is subject to arteriosclerosis and dementia senile with internal destructive processes. The older psychotic will manifest all sorts of excrescences in any part of the body; he is irritable, excitable and volatile. His old age is restless and whilst remaining apparently active, he ends up with tumours.

These are, in brief, the pictures of the miasms. Naturally, it is when the vital imbalance occurs and persists that the characteristics of the miasms set in, in relation to themselves or in conjunction with the others, thereby creating a complete range of symptoms in degrees which are now assessable by radionics or radiesthesia. This assessment, combined with the discovery of other imbalances and the detection of the various chains of cause and effect, opens the way to the speeding up of recovery and the minimising of the chances of relapse.

To summarise briefly, psora is a disequilibrium which is characterised by defects, insufficiencies and inhibitions; it is the change of rhythm in the minus sense, the individual tending towards 'not being', 'not having' and 'not doing', both in mind and body. With syphilis, the disequilibrium reaches the depth of the constant which determines the rhythm of destruction; hence the perverse character recognisable through his covert and overt aggressiveness. Here again, there is a perversion of 'being', 'having' and 'doing'. The psychotic is in a constitutional state resulting from arbitrary or anti-natural suppressions or eliminations; the miasm predisposes the creation of neoformations, thereby confirming its characteristic feature of excess born in the heedless ambition for pleasure. It is the 'must be', 'must have', 'must do', aspect of the tendencies.

ANOTHER OUTLOOK ON AND APPRECIATION OF THE MIASMS

Some readers may not take easily to, or accept completely, the philosophy of homoeopathy and others do not subscribe to radionics, preferring physical or mental radiesthesia. We know that homoeopathic literature presents a complete mosaic of symptoms with the corresponding remedies, and the radionic practitioner as well as the radiesthesist places emphasis upon imbalances. At times these could conflict, and create shadows of doubt. We also know that, with the exception of research workers in both fields, one would be concerned with diagnosis and the administration of treatment. This done, the patient always remains the final judge as to whether he does or does not need further help. However superficial or however deep our investigations of the subject become, we find ourselves constantly overshadowed by the concept of health, with a multitude of considerations arising from past cultures to the present day. Therefore, health is an intellectual concept, the value of which depends on the mental calibre of the individual. Clinically, as well as philosophically, health is discovered to be equated to LIFE.

Life for man implies a beginning and an end, and for a human organism the ultimate goal of death exists at birth. Can we, therefore, imagine life to be a straight line from A to B? Certainly not, since it would imply that nothing decays or suffers imbalances. The line that joins A to B is an oscillating line, showing shocks, counter-shocks and the re-establishment of equilibrium would be the result of all the oscillations of his component parts, namely: cells, tissues, organs, apparatus and the nervous systems.

To understand this oscillating concept, let us examine the cell which is a unity of its own with its electromagnetic dynamic capacity constituted by its positive nucleus negative membrane and neutral protoplasm. When the positive and negative charges are in equilibrium the cell is said to be sane or healthy. In such a case the chemical and physical elements contained in the protoplasm (viz. iron, calcium, phosphates, CI, K, S, etc.) find themselves in a correlated state of balance. Let us now suppose that the electromagnetic charges inducted from the positive nucleus towards the negative membrane can be observed on an oscilloscope. Then we would see the oscillations between the two poles maintaining the said balance.

However, this oscillation is susceptible to influences by external or self-produced agents. If these agents are not in harmony with the existing equilibrium, a disturbance occurs. We must also establish in some way that these oscillations are related to the magnitude and dynamic of the mass, notwithstanding the fact that the size is within the microns range, producing oscillations in the field of micro-frequencies.

The changes of these oscillations can be due to impulses of emotivity, anxiety or frustration acting through reflex mechanisms which activate the circuits of the hypophysis–hypothalamus–suprarenals to discharge the glucocorticoids and the mineral corticoids (this process can be seen in youngsters when blushing and in others in palpitations). This sort of imbalance is instantaneous and will only leave traces on the cells if the impulses producing it become frequent and continuous. In the case of external "aggressions" by bacteria or virus, there is always an attack to try to establish an adequate environment to survive, a sort of symbiosis; the bacteria act externally on the cell and the virus attempt to act internally in the cell, "pretending" to establish an endobiodid. In whatever form, these two have their own intrinsic dynamism and express their own oscillating curves. The contact between the human cell and the germs produces a battle of oscillations. If the cell oscillates dynamically with adequate energy it will override the germ and destroy it; should the germ dynamism be the stronger, the cell will succumb. Whenever the cell wins it remains physically unscarred but will retain in its chemical structure some electro-magnetic influences (or parasites). We could attribute this to the effect of a miasmatic influence.

The viruses infiltrate into the cells, attempting to live as "squatters" (the duration of which could explain the chronic conditions and make clearer Hahnemann's miasms) and to establish a equilibrium with the host cell. Such equilibrium can be upset by any stress that weakens its electromagnetic dynamism and the gate to sickness will be opened. In all cases, the battle is one of electromagnetic balance in which there is, on the one hand, adaptation, and, on the other hand, destruction.

However this process operates, it must be remembered that the elements and trace elements contained in the protoplasm (Fe, Na CI etc.) also have their polarities of + and − functioning. Auguste Lumiere has stated that life is a colloidal equilibrium and its precipitation is death.

Furthermore, all this happens at the level of organic micro-circulation. It is known that the primary purpose of the circulatory system is to bring to the cells the necessary substances for their metabolism and vital regularity, acting also as a channel for elimination to enable the cell to live in a well-maintained environment.

Therefore, the heart, the arteries and the veins are simply conductors of the blood to serve the capillaries to feed the cells. At this precise stage, it would be preferable to think of a functional unity rather than a capillary system. This function is called the "capillary milky way". When it was examined with very special devices it was discovered that the capillary tube is formed like a flat surface of a smooth pavement of flat cells, the walls being .00254mm thick. This structure also covers the other blood vessels and the heart walls. The blood is, therefore, contained in this type of cellular construction. The capillaries have no muscles and cannot contract. But as they nevertheless go through a contracting motion, we can only conclude that these motions are controlled by the rhythm of the electromagnetic oscillations. It is unnecessary to say more about scientific data as we reach the point when we can adopt the electromagnetic concept of life.

Now, if health is deficient, this capillary milky way is also affected in its electromagnetic equilibrium, within some margin of tolerance, to form the basis of the constitutional state of a miasm. Why not conclude that such upset of balance can reach the genes, at any given time, through protein acids which will also be unbalanced in their elicoidal constitution, and produce a miasmatic predisposition on the genetic line. If we are to understand the syphilitic miasm, for example, let us suppose a straight piece of wire with its own polarities maintaining an equilibrium. Then let us break this balance by passing a current through it so as to observe the discharge of the inducted current. Now let us make a wavy pattern with the wire to increase its capacity for induction; and then we can further increase such capacity by twisting it into a spiral. At this stage we are approaching the form of syphilis virus (spirochetes). We have seen the strength and the deep–seated functions of the syphillis miasm in the context of homoeopathic philosophy and we have now observed the same phenomenon in the light of the electromagnetic theory.

This will also explain the success of radionics and radiesthesia assessments of organic functions to detect imbalances that are hardly possible in other forms of diagnosis.

I have, personally, in the light of all this, correlated the electromagnetic interplay of the trace elements with the cells in order to pinpoint the weak spot resulting from some chronic basic disequilibrium. No doubt many readers could investigate these preliminary findings, and I myself hope to find that someone else has already discovered these same connecting links. The deficiencies of the following trace elements are shown by imbalances in the corresponding organs:

Trace element	Organ
Ruthenium	Intestines
Hafnium	Pancreas
Rhodium and Tantalum	Kidneys
Rhenium	Testicles
Lutetium	Bladder
Erbium, Gadolinium, Thulium and Ytterbium	Spleen
Gallium and Indium	Ovaries
Samarium	Thymus
Neodymium	Parathyroid
Praseodymium	Surrenals
Lanthanum	Hypophysis
Yttrium, Columbium, Terbium, Holmium and Dysprosium	Endocrine glands, especially the thyroid

Naturally, these have to be proven on a larger scale of investigation as they are, perhaps, only a beginning.

Before ending, I would like to include another aspect of electromagnetic disturbance due to transitory impulses such as emotions, depression, frustration, guilt, remorse, hate, etc., as they can also affect an individual and his constitution as a whole and may be transmitted to his progeny in their state of imbalance at the moment of procreation. Whether these impulses are transitory or persistent, they nevertheless affect the miasmic condition, perhaps beyond the margin of safety, and if procreation occurs at that moment, the tissue would receive an imprint or engram of the said moment, making it predisposed to the original miasmatic effects. Could this be another answer to explain the predispositon to cancer?

I hope I have now filled some gaps and given food for thought in the direction of better understanding of the various chains of cause and effect we encounter in radionic assessment. Our scales, rates, methods of approach, healing programmes and referring to specialists may or may not have contained this new outlook, but I feel that the more background date we are able to interchange in all fields of healing, in all fields of psychology and in all fields of research and in case histories, the more our methods will be enriched towards achieving greater success with all the friends who have put their trust in us.

CHAPTER THIRTEEN

ALIGNMENT AND POLARISATION

First it is necessary that one recognsises what wrong vibration is, and that one is able to register reaction.

A Treatise on White Magic – Alice Bailey

In previous chapters I have touched once or twice upon the dangers of working in the fields of radionics or radiesthesia, and the exposure this brings at the subtle levels to all manner of energies and forces, some of which may be positively harmful. In any healing practice, orthodox or alternative, the same danger is present and the practitioner is exposed to energies which might harm him. This is more true of radionic work than any other because the auric fields of the practitioner and patient connect, and if there are heavy pathological energies within the patient's field that are potent and filled with highly active energy, they will discharge into the practitioner's field with a rush. If the charge is not so high then the process will be far more insidious. I suspect that every practitioner has experienced the feeling of being shattered after working on a patient at a distance, or following a telephone call during which an intense discussion has taken place about symptoms or some disaster or other.

When you multiply this type of contact with the number of patients handled each day, and take into consideration that the patient load itself consists of people, all of whom have some affliction or other, then you have an energy field consisting of all those unbalanced energies, and you link into that entire field and its contents every time you are contacted by one of them, or when you make an analysis or give treatments. I believe that there is a growing recognition in radionic circles that a very real danger exists, the question is what to do about it?

I suppose the first impulse is to find some sort of protective measure, at the lowest level this is going to comprise of such things as gem mixtures or various other substances, magnets perhaps and I have even seen stickers with magic numbers on them stuck to instrument panels. The next impulse is to build up some sort of protective shell of energy in order to keep the negative influences at bay. Neither of these approaches will solve the problem in the long term.

In *A Treatise on White Magic* this problem is dealt with in great detail from many angles.

Response to wrong vibration will not be basically prevented by the methods of either "building a shell", or by "insulation" through the power of mantrams and visualisation. These two methods are temporary expedients by which those who as yet have something to learn seek to protect themselves. The building of a shell leads to separativeness, as you well know, and necessitates the eventual overcoming of the habit of shell–building, and a shattering and consuming of the shells already built.

To build protective shells is to build barriers that eventually shut out the good as well as the negative influences, and the shells eventually become a prison through which even the transpersonal self cannot penetrate. Protection is arrived at in a number of ways which can be summed up in the words, alignment and polarisation. Now what do I mean by alignment and polarisation?

Alignment is the inner focus of attention on the Self or soul, which must become a constant daily habit. This brings our lower mental body, our astral body and the etheric into alignment. If we are focused in our astral body for example we are not going to be aligned because we will be reacting and coming into resonance with the streams of astral energy that enter our astral field from any number of sources. Alignment with the soul is difficult to reach, and once reached, in the initial stages there is a constant pull from astral energies and activities that are going on around us in the immediate environment or even at a distance.

To understand alignment it helps to go back to the right and left mind–brain model that I outlined in *Radionics: Science or Magic?* The left hemisphere of the brain is used for logical thought processes and the right for intuitive. The right mind–brain can be seen as the higher mind or as St Paul called it 'the mind in Christ' – this is the level of the soul. The lower concrete mind is the carnal mind that Paul spoke of. So if you look at the levels of consciousness, all seven aspects of it you will see these two levels clearly illustrated. In radionic work they have to be aligned, that is they have to be in a reasonable state of resonance and as important, or perhaps even more important the astral and buddhic aspects of the practitioner must be aligned in so far as is possible. Alignment is always bringing the lower bodies into resonance with the higher counterparts, and this can only be done by moving the focus of inner attention from the lower into the higher states of consciousness.

As our chakras are the portals of access to each level, then it should be obvious that they are involved in this process, and the chakras we work through in our radionic work will determine how well protected we are. I will list the rays, planes and chakras to show their correspondences.

RAY	PLANE	QUALITY	CHAKRA
1st ray	Adi	Pure Spirit	Crown
2nd Ray	Anupadaka	Monadic	Heart
3rd ray	Atmic	Will	Throat
4th ray	Buddhic	Intuition	Brow
5th ray	Manasic	Mind	Sacral
6th ray	Astral	Emotion	Solar Plexus
7th ray	Etheric	—	Base

If a practitioner is polarised in their astral body and has a 2nd ray quality governing that body, especially a 6th ray, then they will do most, if not all of their diagnostic work and treatments through the solar plexus. This in itself is a recipe for trouble. If they have several of their bodies and/or personality along the 2nd ray line of energy then sooner or later that practitioner is going to be in all sorts of trouble, due to the fact that they are working at the astral level where most problems arise in terms of physical and psychological health. Their solar plexus/astral focus is like an open doorway through which all of the negative and disease bearing atoms and particles are drawn from the patients they contact at that level.

People with a lot of 2nd ray quality tend to be attracted into one healing art or another, radionics attracts this type of person because of the nature of the work, and many become victims of nervous over-stimulation because they don't even begin to understand what they are involving themselves in. The problem is aggravated by the fact that no one I know who instructs in radionics, understands the dynamics of the problem either, so you get a situation in which the blind are leading the blind. It should be made clear that radionics involves many different energies and only by understanding what they are and acting accordingly will the student evolve, and so transform their inner nature that they will not be distressed by the work. I have said again and again, radionics is more than a form of therapy, it is a means of spiritual development, or can be used as such by those who are aware of the processes and energies involved.

The first step towards creating a safe way of working then, is alignment with the higher aspect of the mental body. This is essential. The next is to work through the brow chakra and not the solar plexus, and please note just what that does. It shifts the focus from the astral plane (solar plexus) to the buddhic plane (brow). This does not mean that anyone working through the brow chakra will be working with buddhic energies, but that is ultimately the goal. The very intention and effort to work through the brow begins to open the way to the higher levels, and on those levels no disease exists. Thus the practitioner can

work in perfect safety and of course with real and far greater effectiveness. This process cannot be taught with words unless those words
come from an instructor who is capable of working from the higher
levels and who has linked certain chakras in a particular manner.

The rays of the practitioner are also of great importance. As I said
previously a lot of energies along the 2nd ray line and the practitioner
will soak up negative energy patterns like a sponge. The paradox is that
the inclusive, intuitive qualities of the 2nd ray are essential to healing
work. A person with little or no 2nd ray qualities cannot heal. So a
balanced ray makeup is vital and it should contain at least one body or
the personality on the 7th ray which is the ray of radionic work, a 5th
ray mind and a 2nd or 6th astral body, provided the virtues of these rays
have been acquired and developed. If the ray makeup is a well balanced
one and the practitioner is polarised in the mental body and can work
through the head and heart chakras, then there is little danger that the
energies and forces of disease within the patient will find a place in their
bodies and the risk of contamination will be minimised or eliminated
altogether.

During the process of daily work in a busy practice it is all too easy to
slip back into old patterns and practitioners may find that the solar
plexus has swung into use, and this is often due to identification with
the problems and needs of the patient. There is a passage in *Esoteric
Healing* which highlights this matter rather nicely.

> One of the major difficulties with which the healer is faced, particularly if
> relatively inexperienced, is the result of this established sympathetic
> relation. There is apt to occur what we might call "transference." The
> healer takes on or takes over the condition of disease or discomfort, not in
> fact but symptomatically. This can incapacitate him or at least intercept
> the free activity of the healing process. It is a glamour and an illusion and
> is based on the healer's achieved capacity to identify himself with his
> patient; it is also founded on his anxiety and great desire to bring relief.
> The healer has become so preoccupied with the patient's need, and so
> decentralised from his own identified and positive consciousness, that
> inadvertently he has become negative and temporarily unprotected.

The text goes on to outline how this problem can be overcome.

> The cure for this, if the healer discovers in himself this tendency, is to
> work through the heart centre as well as the head centre, and thus keep a
> steady flow of the positive energy of love pouring out towards the
> patient. This will insulate him from the disease, but not from the patient.
> He can do this by working through the heart centre within the
> *brahmarandra* (the head centre) and greatly increase the potency of his
> healing work; however, it presupposes a high degree of development on
> the healer's part.

The average healer will not be able to effect this focus in the heart chakra in the crown chakra, but he can work through the head and heart chakras by a deliberate act of will. Eventually when the head and heart chakras are fully linked this method will take on added power and potency.

One of the biggest problems in practice can be the patient who is a sapper, that is an individual who has an innate and often unconscious ability to lock into the practitioner's astral and etheric bodies and siphon off energy. I used to have a real problem with this type of patient, but learned many years ago that the secret of protection lay in correct alignment and polarisation of consciousness. Patients who have this ability can tap into the practitioner over the phone within seconds and in four or five minutes, suck them dry of vitality. One of my patients who used to phone regularly in an attempt to draw energy, found initially that my guard would drop, if when I picked up the phone and made the usual acknowledgement, they remained silent. The silence as you can imagine creates a sort of vacuum into which it is easy to get drawn. I fell for this ploy a couple of times but soon learned to remain silent until they spoke. Sometimes the whole living room would fill with peculiar and chaotic energies as the patient unsuccessfully tried to lock into my solar plexus and astral body.

The purpose of this brief chapter has been to call to your attention in a simple manner, a highly complex problem which can lead to ill health, overstimulation and a deep feeling of fatigue. The cure does not lie in external aids but in the focus of the interior life at the higher levels. Right alignment and polarisation combined with the practice of *harmlessness* will provide full protection from those energies which are inimical to the well-being of the practitioner.

CHAPTER FOURTEEN

RADIONICS AND THE RAY ENERGIES

It should therefore be borne in mind that in this connection we are considering the point of experience where light pours in, bringing revelation, conveying information, evoking the intuition and drawing into the waiting consciousness of the initiate those spiritual laws, those rules of the creative process, those ray conditions and those new energies and forces for which the humanity of any particular period waits, and which are fundamentally needed if the race of men is to move forward into greater spiritual culture and out of the relative darkness in which it at present moves.

DINA Vo. II. Alice Bailey

I suppose it is stating the obvious by repeating again that radionics is a healing art that is directly concerned with energies and forces, and yet few, if any practitioners fully understand the implications and the potential of this fact. After twenty four years study of Bailey's writings and over seventeen years in radionics, I am not even sure that I do, despite the fact that thinking in terms of energy comes to me now with some facility. Since 1972 when *Radionics and the Subtle Anatomy of Man* was first published, I have tended to emphasize this theme, because it is central to our work, and because we have not even begun to tap the potential of radionics. Certainly it has shifted from the relative darkness of its orthodox origins, and is now moving in the right direction encompassing more light as the years go by.

It must be clear to most people that we are in a transitional period in history, and the old Piscean 6th ray order is giving way, albeit a little grudgingly, to the new 7th ray Aquarian one. This shift from one ray to another inevitably brings about chaotic conditions, and heightens resistance to change in those people and institutions who have crystallised into the old and outmoded patterns derived from the 6th ray influence.

My first three books on radionics reflected some basic incoming changes, which most practitioners found little or no difficulty incorporating into their work. These set the stage as far as I was concerned for the more radical shift that was to come. That shift presented itself in *Radionics: Science or Magic?* and the principles outlined in that book caused certain reverberations to run through the community of organised radionics. From some quarters, where crystallised attitudes were most prevalent, there was clear evidence of outright hostility. What I had written threatened the 'establishment' in radionics, and there was something of a backlash which quite frankly surprised me. Where I had expected openness to change and progress, I found individuals in positions of responsibility who could not comprehend what I had outlined in *Radionics: Science or Magic?* and because they did not understand the direction it pointed to, they condemned it. Others were more neutral in their response, but it was obvious, that had I written the book in hieroglyphics it could not have left them more puzzled.

Radionics: Science or Magic? to my mind carries the stream of energy upon which the new radionics will be inaugurated. Like this present volume it signalled its intent to move from Dimension II to Dimension I. It is difficult to describe this phenomena, but I know that the book is already there in that area of consciousness which can be designated as Dimension II. What is more it is already written but not totally fixed or crystallised, in other words the book at that level is a living thing, flexible and open to growth and change. As I write down what is presented to my mind from that level there is a curious tidal flow of ideas, some of them seething with energy which come crashing into consciousness like a heavy wave upon the beach. These frequently turn out to be harbingers of new ideas, or serve to suddenly pull several apparently unrelated factors together in a vital way. In any event there is no question of automatic writing, but simply the effortless presentation of material flowing from one dimension to another. When *Radionics; Science or Magic?* made its appearance I was preparing to quit the field altogether, there were a number of reasons for this, not least amongst them the mass of anomalies present in the system at that time. They still exist of course in the minds of many practitioners but at least *Science or Magic?* held them up for inspection and consideration and hopefully opened the door in a way that would enable creative changes to take place.

Some fifty five hours ago in terms of typing time this book *Chakras – Rays and Radionics,* forcefully announced its presence to my conscious mind. I recognised immediately that this would be my last book on the subject of radionics, and that it would complete my contribution to this field. As it turns out, the material appears to do just that by outlining in as simple a manner as possible the subject of the rays, and indicating how this knowledge can be applied in a practical manner in everyday practise. In some quarters I have been accused of 'riding on the back of radionics' to quote a letter which appeared in the Radionic Quarterly, but in truth I have ridden on the back of knowledge, esoteric knowledge, which is quite legitimate, and by so doing I have deliberately and with firm intent placed radionics in that place of power which will enable future generations of practitioners to unfold its almost unlimited potential.

In *Radionics: Science or Magic?* I wrote of the crisis in radionics which is now running a predictable course. This is a period of crisis in all areas, humanity itself is in a state of crisis so we can expect many changes, but not of course without the shattering of old and outmoded forms. Organised radionics makes an interesting study from the point of view of the ray energies involved. The second, sixth and seventh rays feature very strongly in this healing art, of these the sixth and seventh provide the main energies which give rise to the present crisis. Both energies of course have their positive aspects but in times of crisis the establishment by its very nature tends to try to maintain the status quo, this means that the glamours and vices of these two rays will come into play. The sixth ray will breed crystallised attitudes, divisiveness, partiality, narrow mindedness, possessiveness and rigidity. Factions will arise around personalities who are seeking to serve their own ends under the guise of what is good for radionics.

The group as a whole will lose its wholeness, fragmenting into power structures. The more negative aspects of the seventh ray will bring about the creation of more complex methods of teaching, attempts to mimic the present orthodoxy in the hope of currying favour thus gaining recognition at some future date – a most unlikely event when you consider the rays that govern medicine. Formalism will be accentuated and the rigidity of the sixth ray further enhanced. The writing is on the wall and the energies which will shatter the present form of organised radionics are doing their work.

On the surface this might seem a retrogressive thing, but it is in the nature of progress that crisis precedes the dissipation of old forms. Hopefully a new structure will emerge that will build upon the higher qualities of the energies available. The sixth ray is closely associated with the plane of feeling (the astral plane) whereas the seventh ray relates to the mental levels and brings down the higher forces to anchor them in the everyday world. Sixth ray energy is associated with the solar plexus chakra and emphasises the duality of spirit and form. The seventh ray fosters group unity while the sixth encourages individualism. The keynote of the coming Aquarian age is group consciousness and as those in radionics begin to work with the seventh ray energy, a new and vital group will emerge that reflects the equilibrium and order required in this work. The white magicians who are truly capable of wielding the energies of the rays for healing will be drawn to this field of service. It is interesting to look at some comparisons of sixth and seventh ray energy effects in the light of what is going on in radionics today.

The 6th ray fostered the vision.
The 7th will materialise it.

The 6th ray produced the mystic.
The 7th will produce the white magician.

The 6th ray leads to nationalism. It divides and separates.
The 7th ray leads to fusion and synthesis, blending the energies of spirit and matter.

The 6th ray leads to the formation of groups who function on a personality basis.
The 7th ray produces groups who work in close unison for higher purposes.

The 6th ray brings the sense of duality and physical unity. Materialistic psychology and mechanistic medicine. Therefore the 6th ray in radionics will at this time see progress in aligning itself with the Establishment.
The 7th ray inaugurates a higher fusion.

The 6th ray influence fosters separative instincts, dogmatism, exclusiveness and cults.
The 7th prepares the way for the scientific demonstration of light. Research into melanin in the U.S.A. is already producing some remarkable work with staggering implications for mankind. Ruth Drown always spoke of the energies used in radionics, in terms of light.

As practitioners come to understand the ray energies, they will see that in them is the final piece of the radionic pattern. We will then have:

1. Physical anatomy, physiology and pathology.
2. Subtle bodies.
3. Chakras.
4. The physiology of Light.
5. Pathology as energy imbalance.
6. The Seven Ray energies.
7. A Spiritual Psychology.

These will make radionics into the only true holistic healing art in the world at this time, and place it firmly on the leading edge of the energy sciences.

I can envision the day when suitability to work in the field of radionics will entail a full analysis of the prospective student's subtle bodies, chakras and rays, because the states and nature of these two aspects will largely indicate their suitability or lack of it. Ideally a practitioner should have a good balance of 2nd ray and 1st ray qualities, especially the 7th. Too much 2nd ray influence in an individual's makeup, and they would most likely absorb too much negative energy. On the other hand a prospective practitioner with a lot of 1st ray qualities will be too 'isolated' and not all that effective as a healer.

As the influences of the 6th ray fade out and the 7th takes over a future form of radionics will emerge that will raise this healing art to new heights. New revelations and new technology involving light and electricity will give rise to new instrumentation and open up fresh vistas in radionics. At the same time the profession will attract individuals who through karmic links and inclination will have the power to heal in a most potent manner.

Albert Abrams, Ruth Drown, George and Marjorie De La Warr used the sixth ray to develop and nurture radionics through the first half of this century. Malcom Rae brought his seventh ray influence to bear and from this emerged the concept of geometric patterns and instrumentation to precipitate energies into form. My own contribution utilises the seventh ray through a systematic presentation of the esoteric constitution of man and its relationship to radionic analysis and treatment. The stage has been set, the right energies gathered and set in motion. In a sense this has been a holding action, the seed has been sown from which the new radionics will emerge.

DENTAL FILLINGS AND MERCURY SENSITIVITY
AND
TMJ AND ICV

These two articles appeared in the September 1983 and December 1983 issues of the *Radionic Quarterly*. The are included in order to illustrate how a whole range of apparently unrelated symptoms can so easily arise out of areas of the body, or from factors which may pass unnoticed due to our familiarity with them.

DENTAL FILLINGS AND MERCURY SENSITIVITY

Although having dental cavities filled may not be the most pleasant experience, few, if any of us ever consider that the amalgams used for this purpose might subsequently have a highly detrimental effect upon both our physical and psychological health. Amalgam for filling teeth was first introduced into America in 1825, and into England in 1819, later in 1826 it was used in France. For almost one hundred and thirty five years this substance has been considered basically innocuous until Brazilian dentist Dr Olympio Pinto in his master's thesis, completed in 1959 at Georgetown University in the U.S.A. drew attention to mercury reactions in the human body. By the late 1960's he had advanced the hypothesis that the mercury in mercury-silver amalgam fillings leaches out daily into the body. Today laboratory and clinical evidence shows that this can have a devastating effect on the health of any individual.

Mercury-silver amalgams, commonly called silver amalgams are made up of around 50% mercury and 35% silver, the rest consists of varying amounts of tin, copper and zinc. They are widely used because they are cheaper and easier to use than gold. When the material is placed in the teeth as a filling, electrolysis takes place as saliva reacts with the metal and a corrosive action occurs resulting in a steady release of inorganic mercury which is quickly absorbed into the body. This deposition can be measured by laboratory tests in hair, urine and various body tissues. Mercury-silver amalgams also give off mercury vapours which rapidly traverse lung membranes and enter the blood, they can also diffuse across the blood brain barrier and lodge in the central nervous system. In short mercury–silver fillings in teeth can induce acute and chronic heavy metal poisoning. Later we will look at the symptoms that this form of poisoning can create, but before doing so it is worth considering how certain diseases with unknown or unclear etiology began to appear shortly after mercury–silver amalgams were introduced in 1825. It is a matter of medical history that nephritis was first recognised in 1827 (mercury coincidentally destroys renal tubular epithelium). Hodgkins disease in 1832, leukaemia 1845, Addison's disease 1849, Banti's disease 1881, Gaucher's disease in 1882, anorexia nervosa 1888, Dercum's disease in 1892, Van Jaksch's anaemia in 1890, sickle cell anaemia in 1910, chronic monocytic leukaemia in 1913 and the list goes on.

Mercury poisoning can bring about a multiplicity of symptoms which are usually listed under three basic classifications – neurological, cardiac and immuniologic, most people it seems are more readily affected in their immune system. There is evidence in specific cases that such haematopoetic diseases like Hodgkin's disease and leukaemia were directly attributable to mercury poisoning. A list of mercury amalgam induced symptoms makes disturbing reading, for example, loss of appetite, weight loss, tremor, acute chest and back pain, hyperventilation, anxiety, non-specific flu-like symptoms, thyroid enlargement, high blood pressure, tachycardia, dermatitis, sore throats, swollen glands, swollen and painful joints, fever, malaise, fatigue, burning sensations in the mouth, depression and disturbed sleep. Mercury can corrode the stomach and lining of the duodenum, and as previously mentioned destroy renal epithelium. Clearly it has very unpleasant and far reaching effects both in the physical and psychological spheres.

In America and Canada awareness of mercury poisoning and its subsequent effects on the human mind and body are more wide-spread than anywhere else in the world. The Toxic Element Research Foundation (TERF) issues a quarterly newsletter called *Momentum,* which promotes awareness of the problem of mercury poisoning at a lay and professional level. In these newsletters cases are cited in detail which show conclusively that symptoms can occur as quickly as the day following the filling of cavities, and that people enjoying normal health have literally been devastated overnight to be plagued by bizarre and crippling symptoms until the cause was identified as mercury–silver amalgams. As soon as the amalgams were removed and replaced with non-toxic material the symptoms cleared. One such case involved a teenage girl, she had a 'gone' feeling as soon as her fillings had been put in. Within five months she was suicidal, suffering crippling chest pains, hallucinations, dizziness, hyperventilation, her urine was dark brown and her stools green, she also suffered from dysmenorrhoea and acute anxiety. During that period of time she had been referred to and consulted an internist, a psychiatrist, an allergist, an osteopath, a cardiologist, a minister, a psychologist, a gynaecologist, a chiropractor, a pscyhotherapist, hospital testing and finally a dentist who recognised the cause of the trouble. Within five days of the amalgams being removed she was completely free of all symptoms and back to school, and what is more she remained symptom free.

Another case, this one involving a dental student, showed that his symptoms began five years following insertion of amalgams. He experienced progressive stiffening of his toes, ankles and knees, this progressed to involve his hips, shoulders, fingers and wrists. All tests for arthritis and rheumatoid conditions were negative. Aspirin and stronger drugs were used daily in order to get relief. Within a week of having two fillings removed all symptoms cleared completely. So potent is the mercury poisoning that dentists and their assistants who are involved in removing amalgams have found in retrospect that they have suffered headaches and various other symptoms consistent with the days on which they carried out the work. Hal A. Huggins, D.D.S. points out in an article *Mercury: A Factor in Mental Disease?* that hatters in England who used mercury in the felt hat industry got the shakes and became unstable, hence the term "Mad as a Hatter" and during the American Civil War hatters in Danbury, Connecticut who also used mercury suffered from a condition known as the "Danbury Shakes". In Japan the dumping of mercury waste in the sea resulted in people and cats who ate polluted fish getting neurological diseases. Minamata disease as it was called somewhat resembled multiple sclerosis and many people died from it.

While Radionic Practitioners are well aware of the health problems arising from sensitivity to aluminium poisoning with its effects on the digestive system in particular, and lead poisoning which affects the brain, liver, kidneys, bone marrow and spleen, there is not perhaps such an awareness of the insidious effects arising from the common everyday mercury-silver amalgam used to fill our cavities. It is therefore a point to keep in mind in analysis work and in those cases which do not seem to respond as they should.

TMJ AND ICV

Our modern propensity for abbreviating words can be annoying at times, but in the case of temporomandibular joint and ileocecal valve it can perhaps be forgiven. Both of these parts of the human anatomy when functioning in a balanced manner seldom give us any cause for concern, we daily chew our food and the temporomandibular joint carries out its function; the food passes through the stomach to the small intestine where absorption of nutrients takes place and the waste matter passes on through the ileocecal valve into the large intestine. This of course is how it should be, but when temporomandibular joint dysfunction occurs or the ileocecal valve fails to open or close as it should a whole range of symptoms can occur that apparently have no connection with these areas whatsoever. For this reason both the TMJ and the ICV are of importance to the Radionic practitioner. We pride outselves on determining the cause of disease in the body but how many practitioners would look to the ICV when a patient complained of recurrent flu-like symptoms or bursitis, or to the TMJ when mid-dorsal back pain is the problem? Not many I am sure.

Our body is a very remarkable and complex computer, and I say that without any sense of denigration; it is a most remarkable and beautiful instrument in which unfortunately all too many things can go wrong, and like a computer it may flash a warning signal in the form of symptoms. The body is subjected to constant stimuli from within and without, all of these stimuli are monitored, stored, rejected or retrieved twenty four hours a day by various body systems. Noxious impulses can enter into any system arising from chemical (as we saw in the case of silver-mercury amalgams), physical or mental sources. Even a relatively mild noxious impulse can bring about gross body dysfunction. For example stress will deplete the adrenal glands, this in turn will affect the sartorius/gracilis muscle complex which act as medial stabilisers for the knee and the anterior superior crest of the ilium. Acute knee and sacroiliac pain can result. Foot pronation can cause sciatica or weakness of certain neck muscles, and we are all aware that the gall bladder inflammation creates referred pain in the area of the right scapula. It is a fact that anything can cause problems anywhere in the body, and that the secondary involvement may be very remote from the primary imbalance.

The temporomandibular joint has been of concern to dentists for many years, particularly where patients have clicking jaws, jaw pain and recurrent dislocations. If you place your fingers just in front of your ears and move your jaw you will feel the TMJ articulation. It is hard to believe that such a small joint, and one that we use day in and day out could be a real menace to health when it fails to work properly. The reason, on closer inspection becomes obvious. This small joint has a disproportionate amount of neurologic input in the body computer, in other words a malfunction of the TMJ may involve whole areas of the cerebral cortex, and because of this it can cause disease virtually anywhere in the body. It has been observed time and again that patients with TMJ problems will also often suffer chronic upper back pain, shoulder problems, recurring sacroiliac lesions and intractable headaches along with general poor health. Correction of the TMJ lesion either through dental procedures or chiropractic kinesiology techniques results in the remission of most if not all other symptoms.

While the TMJ lesion is one that we have been aware of due to jaw pain and clicking when eating, or in extremes, dislocation upon yawning, th ileocecal valve syndrome is more occult and less likely to enter our awareness as a specific factor. The ICV is located between the ileum of the small intestine and the caecum of the large intestine. One of its functions is to prevent material in the large intestine from passing back into the small intestine, thus preventing bacteria laden waste products from contaminating this area of the G.I. tract. The other is to keep food products in the small intestine long enough for the digestive processes to be completed.

The ICV syndrome takes two forms, the open and closed. The open form allows waste products that are heavily infected with bacteria to pass back through the valve and into the small intestine so that the individual is likely to be absorbing highly toxic material into the body through the wall of the small intestine. The symptoms that arise from this state of affairs are manifold and mimic many conditons, e.g.:

Headaches	Sudden low back pain
Sudden thirst	Pain around the heart
Faintness	Pseudo sinus infection
Nausea	Pallor
Shoulder pains	Pseudo hypochlorhydria
Dizziness	Dark circles under the eyes
Pseudo bursitis	Tinnitis
Pseudo sacroiliac strain	Flu-like symptoms
Bowel problems	Bursitis

While silver amalgams will create many diverse symptom patterns, the ileocecal valve as a source of trouble cannot be overlooked by the Radionic practitioner who gets a reaction to auto-intoxication. It is in fact one of the most common causes, and one that I, as a chiropractor who uses applied kinesiology frequently come across in daily practice.

The closed or spastic ICV holds back the food that has undergone gastric digestion for too long a period with the result that it becomes toxic and putrid. As these toxins are absorbed any of the above symptoms may begin to make themselves felt. Tense individuals are likely to suffer from closed ICV, and it creates a situation in which they feel unwell if they sleep in. They wake feeling poorly but can at times work it off through activity.

If we find in the course of a radionic analysis that the patient has an ICV problem what can we do? One of the first things is dietary advice, this is absolutely fundamental. The first rule is:

1.   Eliminate *all* roughage from the diet.
2.   Do not eat raw fruit and vegetables.
3.   Eliminate *all* spicy foods.
4.   No alcoholic beverages or liquors.
5.   No caffeine products: coffee, cocoa, chocolate.

These rules should be followed for at least two weeks. Radionic treatment will include detoxification of small intestine and blood; the toning up of the ileocecal valve muscles in the open syndrome and relaxation of the circular muscles of the valve in the closed syndrome. It may be necessary to look for vertebral involvement of L1/L2 or T12. The acupuncture kidney meridian may be involved too. Chlorophyll has proved to be a useful nutritional supplement in ICV open cases and vitamin D, calcium and sometimes silicon in the closed ICV. If ICV cases fail to respond to radionic treatment and the dietary measures outlined above it may be necessary to refer to a practitioner who uses AK (Applied Kinesiology) or Touch for Health techniques, so that direect physical procedures involving neurovascular and neurolymphatic trigger points can be carried out.

I have left any discussion or dealing with TMJ problems until last because there is not a lot that can be done from a radionic point of view, the daily stress of chewing food subjects the TMJ to many physical pressures that cannot be dealt with radionically. If the bite is incorrect then it needs proper correction by dental means and specialist care. Treatment can be given from a supportive role and aimed at increasing the integrity of the fibroelastic tissue of the joint. Arnica, ruta, rhus tox and hypericum may prove useful homoeopathic remedies in such cases, and the diet can be supplemented with manganese and zinc to further aid the joint towards recovery.

Where the practitioner is faced with a patient who exhibits multiple symptom patterns that are more or less chronic, and that have failed to respond to various forms of treatment, it will help to make a point of checking for temporomandibular joint involvement, or the more commonly present open or closed ileocecal valve. We should never underestimate the interconnectedness of all body systems, even the individual teeth themselves. For example through applied kinesiology research it has been found that there is a connection between each tooth and certain muscle groups. The third molar for example represents the psoas muscle which in turn involves the kidney meridian. The central incisor represents the piriformis, adductors and gluteus medius muscles and involves the uterus and seminal vesicles. It may only take an infection or a silver-mercury amalgam filling in the third molar for example, to disturb psoas function which will possibly cause low back problems, or upset the kidney meridian, in which case you get a whole host of symptoms. The moral is, we should never be surprised at what comes up as a causative factor during a radionic analysis, and we should be aware of such factors as the TMJ and ICV syndromes because of the multiple symptom patterns they can throw up when manifesting a state of imbalance.

APPENDIX TWO
DYSBIOSIS

Dysbiosis is the term coined to describe the condition of atypical bacterial flora in the gut. Like amalgam fillings and the ICV and TMJ syndromes, dysbiosis can give rise to many symptoms, which if allowed to persist will quite possibly lead to serious illness later in life.

The normal flora of the gut consists mainly of bacterium bifidum and bacteroides that are anaerobic. E.Coli, enterococci and lactobacilli. These are aerobic and accompany the above. There will also be residual flora in the form of proteus, yeast, aerobic spore producers, clostridia and staphylococci. As long as these remain in a balanced state the intestinal bacteria will do their work properly.

This balance is easily disturbed by antibiotics, antiseptics, and the use of laxatives. Poor nutrition and environmental toxins can also upset the balance. Candida or vaginal thrush is a symptom of dysbiosis and I have seen this make its appearance in a young female patient within seven days of taking a drug to clear acne.

Dysbiosis is a basic illness and is now present all over the world in epidemic proportions. Some of the problems arising from it are:

> Gastric dysfunction
> Constipation or diarrhoea
> Liver, pancreatic and gall bladder dysfunction
> Acne, eczema, allergic illnesses
> Asthma, hay fever
> Sinus problems
> Rheumatism
> Anaemia
> Fatigue
> Depression
> Fungal infections
> Candida
> Nervous exhaustion
> Headaches
> Irritability
> Hypovitaminosis
> Lack of resistance
> Recurrent infections

Dysbiosis has a chain-like reaction which begins in the gut, spreads to the head, then goes to the thorax, quite possibly affecting the heart, then down into the pelvic area where it may disturb ovarian or prostate function. In the later stages it will affect the extremities.

This condition is probably the primary source of auto-intoxication, so it is vital to determine its presence. Once a dysbiosis is cleared, and there are very specific procedures for this, using homoeopathic remedies, then general health will be able to reinstate itself.

FLOW CHART
PROTOCOL FOR RAY–CHAKRA–ORGAN SYSTEM ANALYSIS

1. Determine vitality index
        Physical health index
        Psychological health index
        State of spleen chakra

2. Determine biological age of patient
        Pre–malignancy
        Micro–malignancy
        Macro–malignancy

3. Determine presence of miasms
        Toxins
        Dysbiosis

4. Determine presence of geopathic stress

5. Determine degree of functional integrity of organ systems

6. Determine presence of congestion, overstimulation or lack of co–ordination of mental, astral and etheric bodies

7. Determine states of seven major chakras

8. Determine the transpersonal ray
        the mental body ray
        the astral body ray
        the etheric body ray
        the personality ray

9. Determine which body the transpersonal–self is working through

10. Determine which body the personality is working through

11. Determine the presence of psychic stress

This protocol covers the essential factors in a radionic analysis, practitioners will no doubt have other priorities which can be added to this procedure. For example I would add:

12. Determine transfer flows from lower to higher chakras

RADIONIC ANAYLSIS CHART

This analysis chart is the result of a co–operative effort between astrologer Tad Mann and myself. I supplied one or two ideas and Tad augmented them and designed the chart. The various symbols and patterns utilised are blended to form a pleasing visual impact on one hand, and to provide a practical way to display data regarding the patient's health.

The central feature is the Alembic form or retort which lies within the circle. The top or neck of this alchemical vessel contains the saggital section of the human head and spine, symbol of the path of life, the seven major chakras and a diagram displaying the esoteric constitution of man. The states of the chakras are entered into the vertical pattern, while the ray makeup is displayed in the four circles to the right.

The three sections surrounding the body of the retort carry the names of the various organ systems, the endocrine glands and the seven major chakras. These sections symbolise the triune nature of man and the Monad. Each one tapers into the retort where the energy readings of the organs and chakras are recorded. The upper section containing the three diagrams is extended to emphasise the importance of the Spirit.

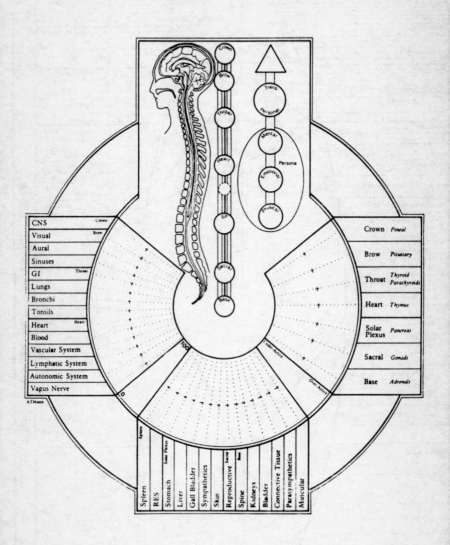

Advanced Radionic Consultants

THE CONSTITUTION OF MAN

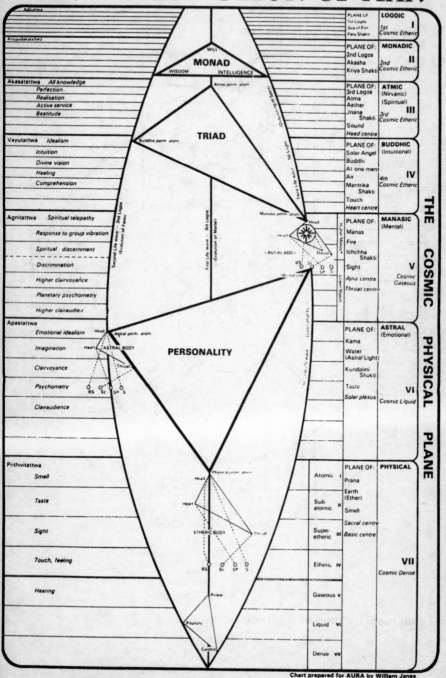

Chart prepared for AURA by William Janes

RADIONIC INSTRUMENTS

TANSLEY RADIONIC M-L FIELD SCANNER.

This compact (32 × 22 × 4½cm) and highly versatile radionic diagnostic and treatment instrument utilises Base 10 and Base 44 modes, and a new and unique system to radionics employing homoeopathic ampules. The latter makes available a level of accuracy and speed not previously obtainable in other systems. The Ampule Mode will appeal directly to the busy practitioner and the beginner alike because of the amplified response which is intrinsically protective and less demanding of the operators own energy fields.

M-L FIELD SCANNER MODULE ONE

Time is of the essence in a busy practice and this module (15 × 22 × 4½cm) is designed to facilitate rapid and accurate analysis of the Rays, Chakras and Subtle Bodies. It is designed also to work in conjunction with the M-L FIELD SCANNER and can be used for diagnosis and treatment; it can however be linked to any radionic instrument.

Both of these new instruments have Interruptor jacks and a smaller jack which enables them to be linked to the Rae Potency Simulator, thus adding to their versatility in everyday practice. The linking wire used between these two sets can also be employed as a chart scanning stylus or remedy selector.

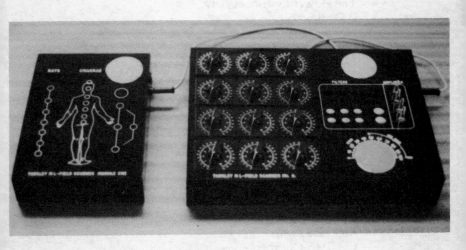

TRAINING SEMINARS IN RADIONICS AND MEDICAL RADIESTHESIA

For details write to:

> Dr David V Tansley, D.C. (U.S.A.)
> Advancd Radionic Consultants,
> 38 South Street,
> Chichester,
> Sussex, England.

SPECIAL SHORT INTENSIVE SEMINARS ARE AVAILABLE TO HEALTH CARE PROFESSIONALS AND OVERSEAS STUDENTS.

For California Flower Essences, write to:

> Earth Spirit Inc.,
> The Flower Essence Society,
> P.O. Box 459,
> Nevada City,
> California 95959,
> U.S.A.

For Flower Essences and Gem Elixirs, write to:

> Pegasus Products Inc.,
> P.O. Box 228,
> Boulder,
> Colorado 80306,
> U.S.A.

For Gem Remedies, write to:

> Ivan J. Ghyssaert,
> Mont De Plan,
> CH–1605 Chexbres,
> Switzerland.

ADVANCED RADIONIC CONSULTANTS

TRAINING SEMINARS

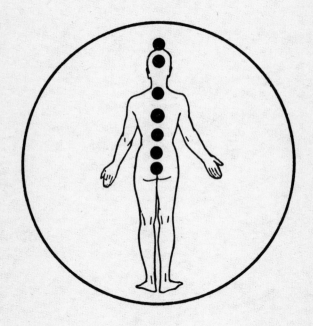

IN

RADIONICS

AND

MEDICAL RADIESTHESIA

— a New Reality in Radionics.